Alzheimer's Disease

Alzheimer's Disease

An Eclipse before Sunset

Dr. A-M. Ghadirian

© 2016 Dr. A-M. Ghadirian

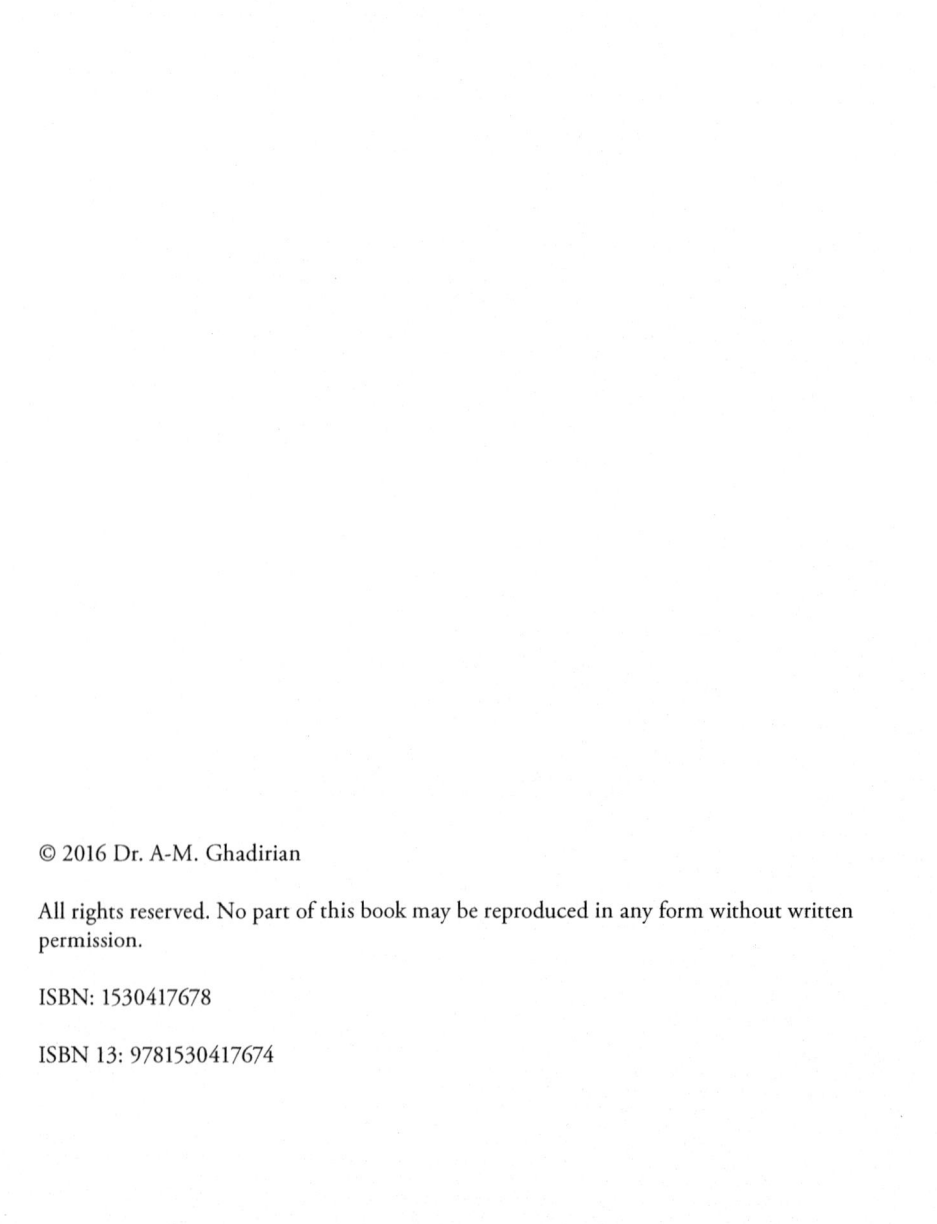

All rights reserved. No part of this book may be reproduced in any form without written permission.

ISBN: 1530417678

ISBN 13: 9781530417674

Table of Contents

Introduction · vii

Aging as a Process · 1
    Modernity and Aging · 3
    Other Aspects of Aging · 6
Understanding Alzheimer's Disease · 8
Alzheimer's Disease in an Aging Society · · · · · · · · · · · · · · · · · · · 12
Biological Dimensions · 17
Psychosocial Dimensions · 22
    Detecting Early Symptoms · 26
    Myths and Misconceptions about Alzheimer's · · · · · · · · · · · · 28
Warning Signs of Alzheimer's Disease · 32
    10 Warning Signs · 33
Risk Factors · 35
    Medical Diseases as Possible Risk Factors · · · · · · · · · · · · · · · · 36
Protective Factors against Alzheimer's Disease · · · · · · · · · · · · · · · 41
    Regular Exercise and Nutrition · 41
    Can diet shield the aging brain? · 42
    Mental and Physical Exercises · 45
    Psychosocial Protective Factors · 46
Memory Changes · 50

Aging and Memory Changes	51
Creativity and Dementia: A Silver Lining	55
Emergence of Musical Abilities in Demented Patients	56
Treatment of Alzheimer's Disease	59
Caring for Patients with Alzheimer's Disease	64
Caring for Elderly Patients: A Family Affair	69
Caring Matters	77
Caring for Caregivers	79
Coping with Caregiver Stress	80
Compassionate Fatigue and Caregivers	82
Spiritual Dimensions	85
The Aging Brain and the Human Soul	87
Some Suggestions on Caring	91
Conclusion	95
References	99
Author Biography	111

Introduction

ALZHEIMER'S DISEASE IS a devastating neurological condition, the incidence of which has been increasing with the rise in the aged population worldwide. Is this the price that modern humanity must pay in exchange for an unprecedented increase in longevity? Is the astonishing progress of science and medicine capable of turning the tide of the prevalence of this disease? Millions of people who hope for long and prosperous lives succumb to an illness toward the end of the journey of their physical existence. This illness attacks their brains and intellect. It is a disease for which there is no cure as of yet, and experts do not agree upon its cause. It progressively strips away layers of memory, the most cherished legacy of human life. As a result, those who suffer from this illness become unable to recognize others—a loved one becomes a stranger; objects, home, and surroundings become incomprehensible. In brief, a life with its memories of people and events vanishes without a trace.

According to the World Health Organization (WHO), it is estimated that between 2000 and 2050, the proportion of the global population over sixty years old will double, from approximately 11 percent to 22 percent—that is to say, from 650 million to 2 billion. (Please see Figure 1.) This rapidly rising number of older people in the world is a cause for celebration, reflecting success on the medical front, not only in decreasing childhood and maternal morbidity but also in prolonging life. On the other hand, this augmentation in the aging population, which deserves care and respect, also poses a challenge to the medical system and to their loved ones, as this phenomenon is accompanied by a consequent increase in the number of those afflicted with Alzheimer's disease. This disease often strikes at around age sixty-five, and there is another sharp increase at age eighty-five. It is estimated that 25–30 percent of people aged eighty-five will develop dementia. Most of these people will suffer from Alzheimer's disease.

With this sea change in the characteristics of society, there is a need to reevaluate the resources and socioeconomic needs of a rising older population in terms of their well-being. The attitude of people toward older generations varies from society to society. In some cultures, the community has high respect for their aged members, whom they view as "elders." In other societies, older people of either gender are tolerated but not especially respected. This variation in attitude is a cause for concern in those suffering from Alzheimer's, who lose their means to defend and protect themselves due to the deterioration of their mental faculties.

This book discusses a number of issues related to Alzheimer's disease and dementia in general for a better understanding of their nature and characteristics. It reviews biological and psychosocial aspects of Alzheimer's disease based on current scientific knowledge and research studies. It also includes a section on spiritual considerations, which are rarely discussed in books on Alzheimer's disease. Such considerations are helpful in broadening our vision and understanding of the nature of the human being and the purpose of life in a holistic way. Furthermore, this book discusses efforts underway to explore a possible cure for this degenerative brain disease and also shares some unconventional remedies for it.

Although the cause of Alzheimer's disease remains an enigma, the book outlines the warning signs as well as the risk factors for this condition. This is followed by a chapter on protective factors against the disease. People often ask questions about how to distinguish memory loss related to Alzheimer's disease from that of normal aging. This issue is discussed in the book. There is also a section on creativity amid dementia—a silver lining—which brings up some very interesting and positive developments that researchers have discovered.

A substantial part of this book is dedicated to the care of Alzheimer's patients, the role and responsibility of caregivers and caring for caregivers, which poses a serious challenge to society. The book offers a number of helpful suggestions for those dealing with this disease.

This work was originally appeared as an article in the *Journal of Baha'i Studies* 1, no. 3. In 1999, it was published in book form by Palabra Publications. The booklet was well received by the public and has been translated and published in French and Persian. The present edition has undergone extensive revision and expansion, and it brings to light new research and knowledge about Alzheimer's.

It is to be noted that this book concentrates more on the psychosocial aspects of Alzheimer's disease and is not intended to be a detailed discussion of its pharmacological treatment, although an overview of this subject is presented. This book is not a substitute for clinical evaluation and treatment by medical experts. Readers should consult their doctors or competent health care professionals on various aspects of the diagnosis, prevention, and treatment of Alzheimer's disease or other dementia.

—A-M. Ghadirian, MD, February 2016

The following is the foreword to the 1999 edition of this work:

Professor Ghadirian's booklet captures the bittersweet experience of Alzheimer's disease. For sufferers, the eclipse is often painfully visible before sunset occurs. For those who support sufferers, the distress is equally intense and even longer lasting.

The dual roles of physicians and, by extension, those who support sufferers of any disease, are to restore functioning and relieve suffering. With Alzheimer's disease, lasting restoration of functioning is presently impossible, but maintenance of remaining function at its best level is feasible through thoughtful structuring of supportive services and, sometimes, medications. Emphasizing what can still be done rather than lamenting the loss of faculties and functions is an appropriate and gratifying goal in Alzheimer's disease. Relieving suffering is done more through care, concern, and empathy for our universal humanness. Professor Ghadirian offers a great deal of helpful guidance. As Francis Weld Peabody said, "The secret of the care of the patient is in caring for the patient."

John H. Griest, MD
Distinguished senior scientist at the Dean Foundation
Clinical professor of psychiatry at the University of Wisconsin Medical School

Aging as a Process

Aging is a lifelong process and not a disease! It is a biological, psychological, social, and spiritual process that we experience during our lives. McPherson identified four types of aging: chronological, biological, psychological, and social.[1] In the chronological sense, aging is counted in years in order to determine rights and legal privileges (e.g., voting, beginning school, retiring, etc.). However, the chronological concept of aging can be deceptive. For example, someone who is thirty years of age may look forty but behave like a twenty-year-old.

Biological aging is determined by internal and external physical changes, such as hormonal changes, development of muscles, the maturation of the reproductive system, and menstrual cycles. While genetics play an important role in this kind of aging, biological changes are also related to our ability to adapt, and they determine our longevity.

Psychological aging refers to the development of and changes in our minds and personalities in areas related to cognition, memory, creativity, learning, and behavior.

Social aging concerns one's perception of others and of the world as well as adaptation to the norms of society. It also includes society's attitude toward the elderly. Social values will determine the extent to which aged individuals will have to deal with loneliness and other challenges and whether they will be supported. Societal structures provide order and stability for the elderly. Culture can influence social aging.

It is thought that these types of aging are not independent from each other but rather interact. For example, a biological aspect of old age might be an impairment of the eyes. This can affect the individual's ability to read or drive a car and will thus limit his or her mobility and lifestyle.[2]

In ancient times, attitudes toward elderly people differed from one culture to another. Although the human life span was much shorter then than at present, nevertheless, in some societies, as people aged, they would lose power and respect, and in some tribes, it was the practice that they be left behind to wither and die.

By contrast, in other societies, old people were considered to be endowed with knowledge and wisdom and were much respected. For example, in the recorded history of the Hebrews, longevity was viewed as a blessing and not a burden. Initially, the Hebrews were nomadic, had large extended families, and were ruled by the eldest male, the patriarch. The patriarch had multiple functions, such as being a religious leader, judge, and teacher. In the Hebrew nomadic culture, old age, particularly in men, was considered to be a sign of wisdom and power.[3]

Among the ancient Greeks, people were afraid of old age; they highly idealized youth, depicting Greek gods with an eternally youthful appearance. Wealth more than old age represented power in society in ancient Greece. Therefore, if an older man was deemed to be powerful, it was mainly because of his wealth.[4]

China has a rich and valuable history of intercultural variation with regard to elderly people. McPherson and others identified three distinct settings with respect to the status of the elderly within the societies of China and Hong Kong: traditional rural villages in mainland China, urban Chinese communities, and the modern industrialized society of Hong Kong (and mainland China). The status of the elderly and the care and respect afforded them in the traditional rural villages continues to be high. The family and the community (in cases where the children have moved out of the village) look after their elderly members. In modernized mainland Chinese cities, there used to be few elderly people, because many would return to their native villages when they reached an advanced age.[5] However, this trend seems to be changing, because, as significant numbers of people have migrated from villages to large cities for jobs and employment, there are fewer younger people left in the countryside to look after the elderly. Like in the Western world, as the number of old people in society rises, caring for the elderly in China remains a challenge, as outlined in another part of this book.

Modernity and Aging

Although with the progress of science and technology, we live longer than we did a hundred years ago, do we really enjoy greater happiness as we age? Since the Industrial Revolution, there has been a shift in society's structure, with people moving from rural areas to urban settings. This shift has changed the landscape of society and people's requirements, needs, and expectations from those of a traditional rural lifestyle to those imposed by life in a city. Moreover, sociopolitical and cultural values of urban life have affected daily life and expectations and have called for new levels of adaptation within different age groups.

Urbanization has brought greater opportunities for education, more working opportunities, better public health, increased medical resources, and improved living conditions, all of which increase longevity. However, this shift in modernization has also been associated with new challenges. For example, the shift from home to factory and migration from rural settlements to life in a large city have adversely affected extended family life and led to the emergence of the nuclear family.[6] The rise of the nuclear family with fewer children, especially in the Western world, has contributed to the isolation of parents and grandparents when they reach old age. Consequently, when a chronic and incapacitating disease such as dementia occurs, there are few offspring available to care for them. In countries such as China, with its one-child policy, the shortage of adult children to care for elderly parents has become more prevalent and a matter of concern (please see section "Caring for Elderly Patients: A Family Affair").

Although it has been argued that modernization leads to the decline in the importance and status of the elderly in society, thoughts are emerging that do not support this notion. In brief, the concept of aging and the status of elderly people vary from culture to culture.

Aging is an existential process; it is part of our nature. Our physical life in this world is not eternal; there is a beginning and an end and a lot to learn and cherish in between. Aging is a universal phenomenon that can be likened to the life of a plant, which begins with a seed, then germinates, grows, and blossoms into flowers. It presents to nature the fruits of its life and then loses its strength and withers. Human aging also has its own seasons from childhood to old age.

If we perceive aging solely in physical terms, we will be happy so long as life allows us the beauty, strength, and fitness to engage in daily activities. With the passage of time, however, the rejuvenation experienced at a younger age fades away, and human beings are beset by chronic diseases and various disabilities. However, in psychological terms, individuals learn from life experience, accumulate wisdom, fulfill potentials, and generally become more mature as they age.

Medicine has improved individual well-being and made longer lifespans possible, but it has not prevented the ravages of old age, such as dementia and loss of memory, the breakdown of metabolic systems, the development of cardiovascular disorders, and many other chronic diseases. Nevertheless, life expectancy has increased at an unprecedented scale. Today people, especially in developed countries can expect to live from 85 to 105 years—or more.

Figure 1

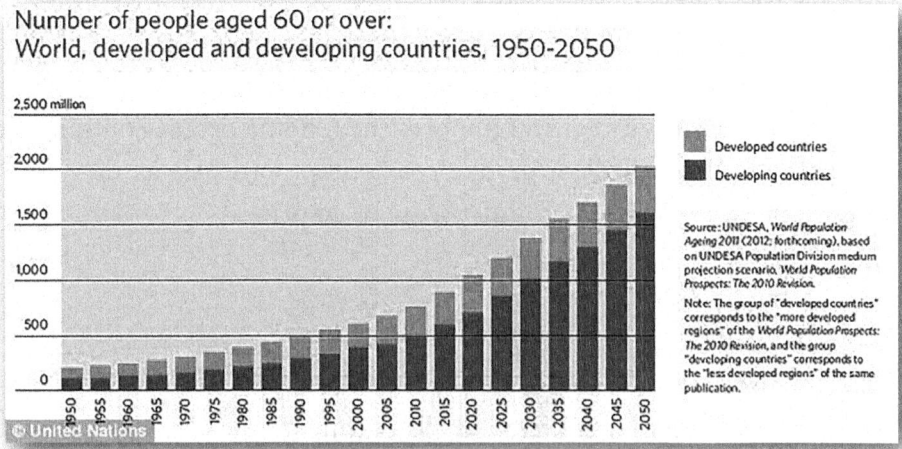

Reprinted with the permission of the United Nations.[7]

By contrast, in ancient times, people did not live beyond twenty or thirty years—forty at most. Consequently, their life-spans were not long enough to allow some of the chronic diseases of the body and brain to appear. People also did not have the knowledge and scientific skill to diagnose dementia and other problems of old age. With the progress of time, knowledge about living longer increased but was confined to a privileged class of people who enjoyed a longer and better quality of life and health care.

Individuals differ from one another in showing signs of aging as well as in their feelings toward this process. Generally, especially in the West, heavy emphasis is placed on physical appearance, and this overidealization of youthful attractiveness has become an obsession that haunts the people in some societies, as the bodily and physical appearance inevitably undergo significant change. Women are more sensitive to this change, and society reinforces it. Cosmetic formulas and aesthetic surgical procedures to maintain youthful beauty and delay the appearance of wrinkles are rampant evidence of the discontent and anxiety they feel, sentiments that feed into a lucrative medical industry that caters to such attitudes.

In such a society where people are so preoccupied, if not obsessed, with external appearance and extrinsic values, the inner beauty and intrinsic values are neglected and impoverished. Some people continue to feel empty and unfulfilled, despite cosmetic procedures, as they find nothing that can satisfy their inner sense of emptiness.

Other Aspects of Aging

With respect to the physiological aspects of aging, one of the symptoms that often brings much angst and dread is the fear of memory loss and dementia, which may result in placement in a nursing home or hospital. Memory and cognitive capacity of the brain, like any other organ of the body, undergo significant change with aging. But not every memory or cognitive change is a sign of a disease such as Alzheimer's. Indeed, there are some individuals in their eighties, nineties, and even in their hundreds who are bright and sharp, and their memory change is not substantial. It is possible that lifestyle, exercise, nutrition, and fewer medical illnesses are some factors that enable these individuals to arrive at an advanced age in such a condition.

Besides the psychological, biological, and social aspects of the human aging process, there is another dimension that is rarely discussed in the academic literature on aging and Alzheimer's—the spiritual dimension, which is briefly presented here.

Spirituality is closely related to the purpose and meaning of aging in the journey through this world. Aging is a developmental expression of the human body and mind. The body is the temple of the soul, and the soul is eternal, while the mind and body are mortal. Through the spiritual dimension of aging, we can perceive that the purpose of the body is to accompany the soul during its existence on this physical plane. "The spiritual evolution of man does not follow the material pattern of ascent and decline. Whereas in the latter a period of growth is followed by decline and eventual death, in the former no such decline or death occurs. Although the extent of this progress varies from one individual to another, the soul maintains a continuous course of advancement."[8] Family members and patients who have a spiritual perspective on life are more likely to accept the reality of an illness and relate to the patient with compassion and understanding, a subject that will be discussed in a later chapter of this book on caring for patients with Alzheimer's.

Understanding Alzheimer's Disease

Consider how the human intellect develops and weakens,
and may at times come to naught, whereas the soul changeth not.

—'Abdu'l-Bahá

Alzheimer's disease, a form of dementia, has been increasing in prevalence across the globe. As this rise is closely related to the increase in the world's aging population, it will be useful to briefly review the phenomenon of the rapid increase of elderly people before elaborating on Alzheimer's disease.

Aging is a natural process of life. It is not a disease, although as age increases, a number of illnesses less frequent in younger individuals may appear. Aging is one of the most important social phenomena of our time. This rise in the aging population will bring changes to the sociocultural landscape of society and will present new challenges to meet the medical, mental-health, and economic needs of this population. In a world where being young and beautiful is overidealized, advanced age is not welcomed as another season of life to look forward to.

As the aging population rises, it is estimated that within a few years, the number of people aged sixty-five and older will outnumber children under age five. Factors that contribute to this demographic change are a decrease in birthrate and a significant increase in life expectancy, which continues to accelerate.[9]

Figure 2
Young Children and Older People as a Percentage of Global Population: 1950–2050

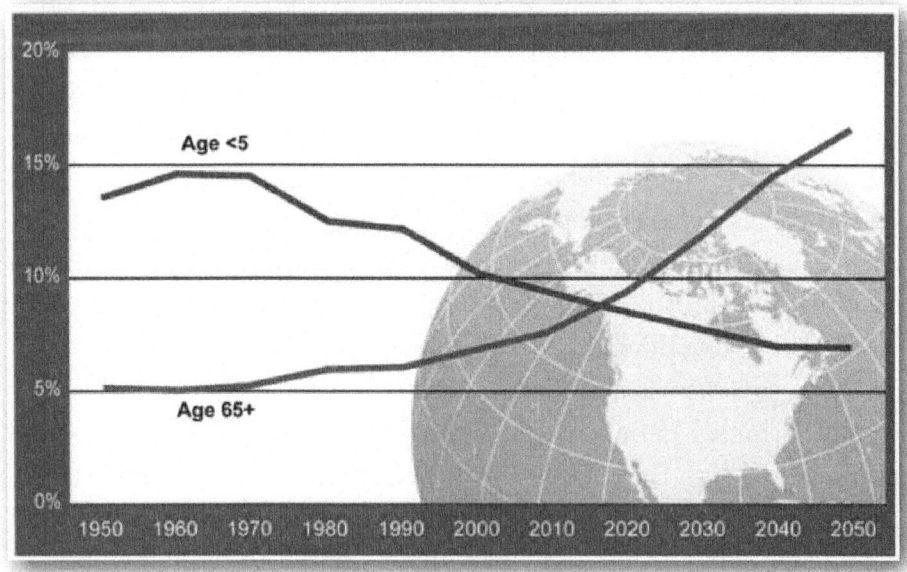

With permission from United Nations Publications, New York, NY.[10]

Since the beginning of the twentieth century, there has been a shift in the leading causes of disease and death in the world's population. At the start of that century, the major causes of mortality were infections and related diseases, especially among young children. The trend has changed significantly since then, and currently, in developing countries, chronic, noncommunicable (not infectious) diseases, such as heart disease, cancer, and diabetes, are the major threats to life in adults, young and old. These illnesses are related to changes that have occurred in modern times, such as lack of sufficient exercise, a sedentary lifestyle, unhealthy eating habits, the rise of obesity, and other factors in addition to aging. Such diseases will impose a heavy economic burden on society.[11]

With the decline of the death rate among older people, it is expected that the number of those aged eighty and older will rise rapidly, and consequently, more people will live past one hundred years. On the other hand, the health of the older population will be hampered by a rise in dementia and Alzheimer's disease (in addition to the maladies mentioned above). So although seniors may potentially lead active and enjoyable lives into old age, consideration must also be given to the possibility that they may face the daunting and serious consequences of illnesses later in life. As mentioned above, it has been estimated that 25–30 percent of the population aged eighty-five or older will experience dementia, including Alzheimer's. Unless an effective prevention and treatment are found for this illness, its prevalence in an aging population will rise worldwide.[12]

Although there is no effective treatment for Alzheimer's disease, nor is there a highly definitive and well-established means for its prevention, nevertheless, there have been growing numbers of research studies, programs, and diversified procedures and efforts, from nutrition and herbal substances to exercises that aim to prevent or delay the onset of this debilitating disease of the brain.

Caring for Alzheimer's patients is a daunting task that requires much patience and a profound sense of empathy as well as compassion and love for the person suffering from the disease. It is important for the caregiver not to become dismayed or disheartened by the disturbing behavior of the Alzheimer's sufferer, as the disease stems from the degeneration of the brain. In such a situation, the caregiver's devotion will be tested because, although caregiving is one of the noblest of human activities, to face a loved one who has turned into a hurtful stranger is a heart-rending experience. Maintaining a positive attitude, one filled with loving compassion, is a formidable task. In such circumstances, caregivers need to realize that it is the disease that causes the unpleasant behavior. This is not to deny that, for example, when a husband sees his wife drifting into forgetfulness, indifference, and rejection, it is normal that he feel sadness for the loss of a lifelong relationship of love. However, it is also to be noted that between these episodes of belligerence and accusatory behavior, there are also moments of gentle kindness and calm.

Alzheimer's Disease in an Aging Society

When Alois Alzheimer, a German neurologist and psychiatrist, discovered this disease in 1906, he initially noted that it was a form of accelerated aging. He described a middle-aged patient who had developed symptoms of dementia with deterioration of memory, language, and behavior. The patient died at age fifty-five, and an analysis of her brain tissue after death showed degenerative plaques. The illness was considered a presenile dementia until the 1960s, when plaques of degenerated neuronal cells (neurofibrillary tangles) in the brain were noted to be correlated to Alzheimer's disease.[13]

Alzheimer's disease is the most common form of dementia, which is a general term for mental and neurocognitive disorders with loss of memory and other cognitive and behavioral symptoms mentioned above. Dementia is defined as a clinical illness that is characterized by "the development of multiple cognitive deficits that are severe enough to interfere with daily functioning."[14] However, Alzheimer's involves more than loss of memory. With the progress of the illness comes confusion, intellectual deterioration, impairment of judgment, changes of mood and personality, and disturbance of orientation and concentration. It is a degenerative disease of the brain cells and accounts for more than 50 percent of all dementia patients.[15] Agitation, anger, and mistrust of friends and strangers make it hard for caregivers to serve these patients.

There are many forms of dementia that are usually associated with a decline in intellectual and cognitive function, with changes in behavior and impairment of social activities. Dementias other than Alzheimer's can be caused by medical diseases such as cerebrovascular diseases, infectious diseases, endocrine disorders like diabetes, and others.[16] These dementias include frontotemporal dementia, dementia due to consumption of toxic substances, and vascular dementia. Vascular dementia is a type of dementia with impairment of cognitive function due to disorders of blood circulation of the brain as a result of cardiovascular and related diseases. The focus of this book is primarily on Alzheimer-type dementia.

According to the definition of the American Psychiatric Association, the diagnosis of dementia is based on the following symptoms: (1) demonstrable evidence of impairment in short-term memory with inability to learn new information and impairment in long-term memory with inability to recall information that was known in the past; (2) impairment in abstract thinking, characterized by the inability to find similarities and differences between related words and their meanings; (3) impaired judgment and disturbances of higher cortical (brain) function; and (4) personality changes and disturbances that significantly interfere with work, usual social activities, or relationships with others.[17]

As the aged population increases, it is expected that the number of Alzheimer's patients will also rise. It has been estimated that the number of Americans aged sixty-five and over, which totaled forty-three million in 2012, will increase to approximately eighty-four million by 2050 (from 14 percent to 21 percent of the population, respectively). Moreover, according to the University of Southern California, between 2010 and 2050, there will be a significant increase of 153 percent in the number of people seventy years and older with Alzheimer's disease.[18]

Experts in the field have reported that there are presently 33.9 million people in the world who suffer from Alzheimer's disease. The prevalence of this disease is expected to triple by 2050.[19] In Canada alone, it was estimated that in 2008, over 480,000 Canadians were affected by this disease. [20] The cost of dementia in Canada will more than double every ten years from $15 billion in 2008 to $153 billion in 2038.

Based on a Lancet report (2005), the global prevalence of dementia was "estimated to be 3.9 percent in people 60+ years with the regional prevalence being 1.6 percent in Africa, 4.0 percent in China and Western Pacific regions, 4.6 percent in Latin America, 5.4 percent in Western Europe and 6.4 percent in North America."[21]

Figure 3 shows the prevalence of dementia in some parts of the world.[22]

Figure 3

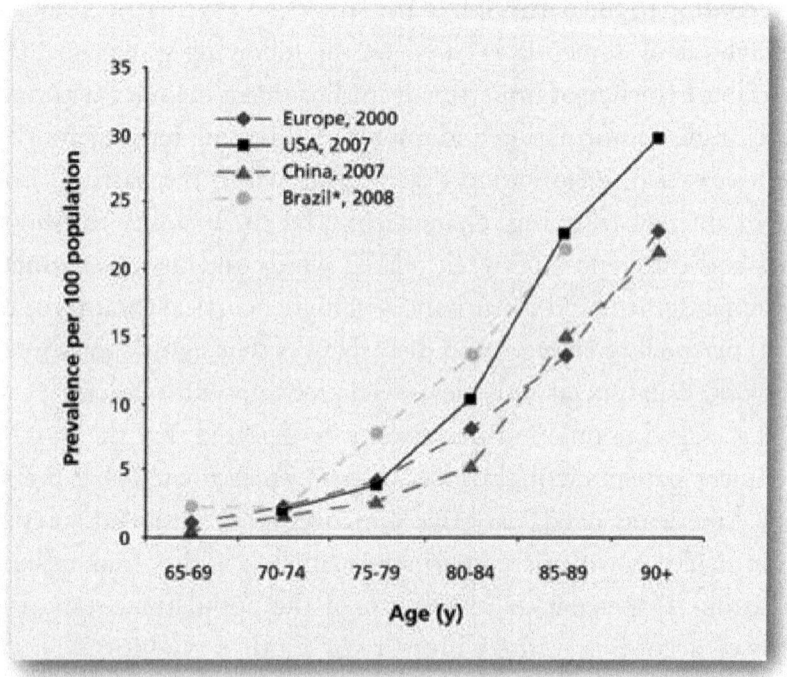

Age-specific incidence of Alzheimer's disease (per 1 000 person years) across continents and countries.*, incidence of all types of dementia

Reproduced with permission of Les Laboratoires Servier. Qui C et al., 2009. Copyright © Les Laboratoires 2009.

Although symptoms of Alzheimer's may vary from person to person, the most common initial one is memory decline, notably gradual worsening of the ability to remember new information and recent events. With the passage of time, this becomes increasingly worrisome. As Nobel Prize winner Eric Kandel stated, "Memory is the glue that holds our mental life together. Without memory each moment in life is an isolated fragment."[23] As Alzheimer's disease progresses, the initial symptoms of forgetfulness and other cognitive impairments are followed by behavioral and language deterioration, including that of communication, coordination in walking, difficulty in dressing, and other matters of self-management. Eventually sufferers become totally dependent on the help of others and are unable to interact with people around them. The more the deterioration of mental and physical activities of the Alzheimer's patient advances, the more challenging the task and responsibility of caregivers and, hence, their level of stress and fatigue. The National Institute on Aging outlined three stages in the development of Alzheimer's disease, the brief high points of which are as follows:

Mild stage of Alzheimer's disease: In this stage, the symptoms of cognitive decline associated with forgetfulness and memory loss become evident. Patients repeat the same questions. They get lost easily, show poor judgement, and take longer to complete routine daily tasks. Mood and personality changes may become apparent. According to the National Institute on Aging, individuals are often diagnosed with Alzheimer's disease during this stage.

Moderate stage: As the disease progresses, the patient's reasoning, thought, and control of language are adversely affected, and cognitive function further deteriorates. Confusion may prevail, and patients may not be able to recognize their family or friends. They may not be capable of learning new things or carrying out daily tasks like getting dressed. In this stage, patients may experience delusions, hallucinations, and paranoid thoughts.

Severe stage: In this stage, degenerative plaques will have spread, and the brain becomes atrophied. Patients in this final stage are unable to communicate and are totally dependent on the nurse or caregiver for care. Toward the end, they likely become bedridden.[24]

Although dementia is reported to be one of the leading causes of death in older people, this cause has largely been underreported, even when it was associated with other medical disorders.[25]

Biological Dimensions

The biological cause of this illness is not clearly known, but some possible contributing factors have been identified. Age appears to be the most important factor, and aging of the brain is being carefully studied. Genetic predisposition is also an important factor, for the illness is more prevalent in certain families. There is a higher prevalence of the illness among women, but it remains to be seen whether this is because of a greater longevity and higher number of older women in society as compared with men or whether it is due to some as yet unrecognized hormonal and environmental changes in the lives of women. [26]

A number of theories on the cause of Alzheimer's disease—viral infection, aluminum toxicity, chromosomal abnormalities, cerebrovascular amyloidosis, immunological deficiencies, and deficits in the cholinergic system of the brain—have been proposed, but none has been definitively proven. It is possible that the disease is not caused by a single factor but rather by a combination of factors or an accumulation of insults to the brain. In fact, there are also subtypes of Alzheimer's disease.

Although there has been significant scientific progress in understanding neurodegenerative diseases such as Alzheimer's, science is still exploring the ways that they develop. For example, research scientists have discovered that some neurodegenerative diseases are caused by the malformation or incorrect folding of protein in the brain. Recent research studies reveal that the misfolded proteins may underlie a possible transmission of Alzheimer's disease from person to person through medical procedures. For example, it is possible that through medical procedures such as neurosurgery or medical transplants, the beta-amyloid seeds responsible for Alzheimer's could be transmitted from one person to another.[27] However, much research and reliable evidence would be required to validate this hypothesis. Moreover, beta-amyloid is not the only causative factor for developing Alzheimer's.

Harvard neuroscientist Randy Buckner studied normal memory during aging with interesting findings. As we age, our skin, muscles, bones, and other body parts will change, and so it is with the brain. As the brain changes, memory and cognitive function also decline. Using special brain images (fMRIs), Bruckner compared brain function of healthy young individuals with that of healthy older adults. Participants in the study were asked to memorize a series of words. Their brains were then scanned when they recalled the words. Although one might expect less brain activity in older adults, it was noted in this study that there was an increase of it. It is suggested that this increased brain activity was probably a form of compensation as the older brain was trying to work harder in order to perform as close to a normal level as possible.[28]

David Bennett of the Rush University Alzheimer's Disease Center in Chicago studied the brains of Alzheimer's patients extensively. He reported that the brain of a ninety-year-old nun who had shown no decline in her cognitive performance during her life manifested substantial amounts of beta-amyloid plaques when examined in an autopsy after her death. He was very intrigued by this observation and wondered how she could have had so much beta-amyloid in her brain without experiencing memory deficit.[29]

Many researchers believe that beta-amyloid accumulation in the brain is responsible for Alzheimer's disease. They also believe that the brains of people like the above individual have a kind of "cognitive reserve," which enables some of them to function well in spite of damage caused by plaques in the brain.[30] The matter of the efficient functioning of the brain as a result of cognitive reserve to draw upon for compensation when diseases such as Alzheimer's develop is a new focus of debate and research exploration. Is cognitive reserve more pronounced in those who have larger brains with more brain cells so that if some cells die due to disease, other cells can compensate? This hypothesis has not been proven. Rather, based on brain-imagery studies, there is compelling evidence that "brain efficiency, not size, underlies cognitive capacity."[31] Therefore, it is believed that the cognitive reserve of the brain depends on the brain's efficiency and its operation (e.g., when the damaged cells are blocking neuronal activities, the brain uses "alternative routes"[32] to restore and rewire itself and perform in the face of cognitive tests).

As the brain ages, there is a continuous loss of brain cells, which ultimately reduces brain volume; this is a normal part of the aging process. Heavy drinking of alcohol can contribute to additional loss of brain cells. The death of neurons (brain cells), which impacts memory as well, is a very slow process. More important than the loss of neurons is the loss of synapses, points where nervous impulses are transmitted from one neuron to another and which facilitate communication between neurons. Loss of synapses leads to dysfunction of neuronal cells, and this phenomenon is accelerated with the onset of dementia, including Alzheimer's disease.[33]

According to Norman Doidge, with the advancement of age comes a reorganization within the brain to compensate for losses. This capacity of the brain to readjust its structure to compensate for deterioration is due to its plasticity. The cognitive function of the brain may be maintained through neurogenesis (the growth and development of nervous tissue), even to a limited extent, in old age. Consequently, some of the brain activities are shifted from one lobe to the other.[34]

While in the normal process of aging, there is a loss of the larger neurons (nerve cells) of the brain, in patients suffering from dementia, particularly of the Alzheimer's type, there are numerous plaques of degenerated neuronal cells (neurofibrillary tangles) in the hippocampus and cortical regions. Depending on the locality of areas affected, symptoms of Alzheimer's may vary from person to person. The appearance of these amyloid plaques in the dominant or nondominant hemisphere of the brain can make a difference in the symptoms of Alzheimer's due to the asymmetry of brain function. For example, if the damage occurs in the limbic system of the brain, it may cause memory deficits, including difficulty in finding objects and remembering where they were placed. These patients may also become suspicious and exhibit changes in mood and emotion (e.g., anxiety, depression, or aggression).

If the temporal lobes of the brain show degenerative plaques, learning new things and short-term memory will be affected, while if the hippocampus area is affected, remembering words as well as verbal and visual memories may become disrupted. Consequently, patients become forgetful of recent events, can't articulate words, and are unable to recognize familiar objects, faces, or places.

Likewise, when other lobes of the brain are damaged, other signs and symptoms will appear, such as changes in judgement, difficulty in organizing activities, inability to express ideas clearly, getting lost easily, and behavioral changes, such as becoming disinterested and withdrawing from others or repeating an activity over and over. [35]

The degenerative destruction caused by Alzheimer's disease is likened to the erasure of the hard drive of a computer "beginning with the most recent files and working backwards. An initial sign of the disease is often the failure to recall events of the past few days...As the illness progresses, however, the old as well as the new memories gradually disappear until even loved ones are no longer recognized."[36] In contrast to the computer in this analogy, one cannot reboot the human brain and reload the files or programs. In fact, Alzheimer's disease not only erases information, "it destroys the very hardware of the brain, which is composed of more than 100 billion nerve cells [neurons] with 100 trillion connections among them."[37]

Recent research studies of patients with dementia show that some previously acquired talents and skills may remain unaffected, in spite of the neurological impairment due to dementia. It is reported that some of these patients demonstrate musical skills and artistic abilities such as painting. In one case, a businessman who developed dementia demonstrated artistic ability to paint after the onset of the disease. Strangely, his painting work steadily improved despite his cognitive deterioration. In another instance, the artistic ability and productivity of a patient with Alzheimer's disease continued unabated in spite of mental deterioration. Although this unexpected development is rare in Alzheimer's patients and difficult to explain, it is possible that, in these cases, the plaques that were the cause of degeneration had not affected the right hemisphere of the brain, or perhaps the dementia had not destroyed all mental functions.[38]

Psychosocial Dimensions

It appears that science and technology have paved the way for the rise of an aging population before the human mind and soul are prepared to cope with all the physical, psychological, social, and spiritual consequences of this development. At a time when we are unraveling the mysteries of the universe and conquering nature to our advantage, we face one of our worst fears—the fear of losing our intelligence and memory.

Loss of conscious awareness and the intellectual ability to appraise life circumstances and to maintain a dynamic and effective relationship with the world around us can be overwhelming, particularly at a time when, due to age, our physical and psychological strength is declining. The power of understanding is described as the most valuable asset of human reality. The loss of this power presents itself like a monster at the end of the human journey or an eclipse before sunset.

The tragic impact of Alzheimer's disease affects not only the victim but also the relatives, who find a loved one slowly descending into confusion and oblivion or turning into a mistrustful and belligerent stranger in their midst. One patient with Alzheimer's disease was unable to remember that each night, she would get up and go to the refrigerator for a snack. In the morning, she would accuse others in the house of stealing her food. For the caregivers, living with such an individual is a test of tolerance, patience, and love, particularly if they don't know the vicissitudes of the illness.

Patients with Alzheimer's disease show their symptoms in different ways according to their personality structure and the extent of their illness. It is believed that Alzheimer's disease progresses more rapidly when it appears in middle-aged people. In general, after discovering that they are losing their memory, a process over which they have no control, patients may experience a sense of helplessness and despair.

In the early stage of Alzheimer's, many patients have a sense of shame due to the fact that their memory is fading away. They may try to hide this deficiency. Some wonder if this illness is worse than others, such as cancer. In the film *Still Alice* (2015), Julianne Moore magnificently plays the role of an Alzheimer's patient facing this dreadful plight. At one point, she cries out "I wish I had cancer. I wouldn't feel so ashamed." What frightens her deeply is learning that she may have passed the gene on to her children and, eventually, to her future grandchildren. "This is hell—but it gets worse," she says.[39]

As the disease progresses to the next stage, patients express considerable mistrust and anger—a protest against what they have lost. Loved ones can no longer be trusted or sometimes even recognized, and home is no longer home. Life becomes very lonesome as they withdraw into a state of total resignation and progressively slip into a dark world of oblivion. At times a lucid, presence of mind and clear memory may reappear, but like the rays of the sun piercing through a dense cloud, these are sparse and momentary. As the illness progresses further, patients eventually move toward a vegetative state in which they become entirely dependent on others for their survival.

Imagine the brain as a house full of lights in which someone begins turning them off, one by one. There will come a time when the entire house is in darkness. The development of Alzheimer's disease with progressive erosion of memory is like the turning off of the lights of memories together with all the emotions, ideas, and history of the past.[40] In such a darkened house, it is hard to recognize people, including loved ones, and it is not possible to switch the lights back on.

Sometimes patients may be totally confused and, in some cases, hallucinate or experience delusions and agitation. They may complain bitterly of being persecuted. Their behavior may become inappropriate, entirely contrary to their personal values, and hence, a great embarrassment to their family. They may speak to people who are not present and who, in fact, may have died years ago. They may misidentify strange people as their relatives and reject some of their loved ones, perceived as their enemies or imposters pretending to be their friends or family in order to take advantage of them.

In patients with dementia, including Alzheimer's, behavioral problems worsen during the evening. Their fear and anxiety increase, and they tend to be more confused and lost at night. That darkness is associated with fear and could be partly due to problems with cataracts or other visual impairment of old age, but often it could be due to insecurity caused by mental confusion or the anguish of being lost or abandoned. Wandering can be a serious problem and may increase at night because of restlessness and disorientation. However, there are other factors, such as moving to a new and unfamiliar place, that may cause a patient to wander. Sometimes wandering may be aimless without a discernable reason and is usually due to impairment of brain function. Special attention should be given to patients who might wander in an agitated state.

People with Alzheimer's disease are very sensitive to rejection; in fact, symptoms of mistrustfulness may serve as a defense against rejection. As a result of fear of loss of control over themselves and their possessions, demented patients may decide to protect their belongings by hiding them. When they fail to find what they have hidden, they suspect others, usually the closest relative or friend, as the culprit. It is very painful for a loved one to be accused of wrongdoing and yet maintain a loving and caring relationship with such a patient. But this is the very challenge that family members and caregivers face, as most of the mistrustful ideations are consequences of memory loss and symptoms of the illness, such as paranoid thinking.

Alzheimer's patients often have precious memories of the past, which, before these memories fade away, need to be captured and treasured by their loved ones. These may include wonderful stories and insightful experiences, some of which were never shared before and with the passage of time, will be erased forever. We should always be mindful of the fact that behind the disease is a person with a soul, who used to be, for example, very kind and generous, but is now confused or bewildered. He or she deserves compassionate care and love as a human being. The initial stage of the illness, when the patient still has some awareness of his or her situation, can be frightening to the patient. The most penetrating fear is the fear of being abandoned and of losing control over one's self, which can lead to utter hopelessness. It is different from losing a leg, where a person is still able to develop a strategy and cope or seek the advice of an expert to manage the situation.

Inability of Alzheimer's patients to recognize family members or friends is not simply because of vision problems but rather, more importantly, is due to the effect of the degeneration of brain cells, which makes it difficult to remember and recognize. This is also a reason that a spouse or relative is misidentified as a stranger. In these circumstances, it is possible that the ability to properly assemble relevant information in order to recognize the individual or object has been lost. This phenomenon is called *agnosia*, a Latin word meaning "to not know."[41] A typical example is that of a man coming home from work and his wife telling him at the door that he is not her husband. She may admit that he looks like her husband but insists that he is not her real husband or believes that he is an imposter. Her brain is unable to interpret the image she sees in front of her as being compatible with the one she has stored in her memory. Reassurance may help to solve the problem. But confrontation and argument usually worsen the situation. Sometimes a patient may speak about expecting the arrival of someone who died many years ago. One interpretation of this behavior is that perhaps, in their mind, "the past has become the present."[42]

Detecting Early Symptoms

Discovering the early symptoms of this degenerative disease is vital, but accomplishing this task is very difficult. Since 1980, progress in medical science and technology has made it possible to discover ways of gaining some knowledge regarding how to detect the disease, but recognition of very early symptoms still remains elusive.

One of the most common symptoms that comes to the attention of the patient and close family members is a decline in cognitive memory. But when forgetfulness appears, the disease is already in progress. Nevertheless, during the past thirty years, specialized neuropsychological (cognitive) tests conducted by well-qualified experts have yielded valuable results. These tests, however, are based on symptoms of cognitive decline that are underway, and the definitive diagnosis is very time consuming.

Another approach that is very promising is the use of magnetic resonance imaging (MRI) and functional MRI (fMRI), which measures brain activities during the performance of a cognitive task. Also, positron emission tomography (PET) has transformed scientific research for an evidence-based diagnosis of Alzheimer's. By tracking the beta-amyloid concentration in the brain and the progress of this disease, physicians can monitor the patient's response to new medication.[43] In addition, because of the neurotoxic effects of beta-amyloid, recent research studies have been exploring a way to inhibit or block the formation of this substance.[44] In view of the fact that the theory of beta-amyloid is one of several theories of the cause of Alzheimer's, the above approaches will serve one concept of etiology.

Aside from the above neuropsychological tests and those through fMRI and PET, there is another approach that is quite different but valuable—the observation of family members, colleagues, or friends of an individual with potential Alzheimer's who is experiencing some symptoms of memory deficit. Although cognitive decline is not the only symptom of Alzheimer's, it is the most consistent and prevalent one for this disease.

Among family members, the spouse and adult children as well as close friends of the patient play a very important role in observation not only of decline in memory but also of changes in performance and behavior of someone with potential Alzheimer's disease. The spouse, other close family members, and friends have greater insight and knowledge of behavioral patterns of the person from the past to the present.

According to the American Academy of Neurology (AAN), loss of recent memory, which is called short-term memory, is usually the earliest warning symptom of Alzheimer's. Repetition of certain words or stories is another early indicator. But the process of development of the disease is often so slow and gradual in the early stage that it may not be recognized.[45]

Why is detecting the initial signs and symptoms so important? Aside from early intervention and treatment (even though presently, effective treatment is lacking), there are social and legal implications in such areas as finalizing business projects, writing a will and dividing one's inheritance with clarity of thought, and many other important decisions. A diagnosis of Alzheimer's disease may cause a person's mental competence to be questioned as well as his or her ability to make sound and well-informed decisions.

As Alzheimer's disease is a progressively degenerative disease, it is important to do the necessary evaluation as soon as possible to avoid problems later, when the person with Alzheimer's may not be able to participate with a sound mind in decision-making processes. "Many matters can be arranged in advance of the disease's more debilitating phase. Does the individual have a durable power of attorney? Who will she assign that to? Should she continue to live in her home or should she choose an alternative? What about driving? Is there a need to supervise medications? Who will manage her financial matters? This is the time when she and her family can decide these things, rather than waiting until a guardian must be appointed to speak for her."[46] One woman came to see her doctor accompanied by her adult son. He expressed a concern about her by telling the doctor that his mother was constantly unplugging electrical devices and also her phone line. He wondered how he would be able to contact her to find out how she was because of what she did. He found these changes in her behavior to be alarming. She was later diagnosed to be at a relatively early stage of Alzheimer's.[47]

Myths and Misconceptions about Alzheimer's

There are a number of misconceptions in the general population about Alzheimer's disease. One of the most common is that it is a disease of old age. Although the majority of patients suffering from Alzheimer's are over sixty-five years of age, this illness can afflict individuals younger than sixty-five—even those who are in their thirties, forties, and fifties. When this occurs, the disease is called early-onset or younger-onset Alzheimer's, and these patients comprise about 5 percent of those suffering from Alzheimer's disease. There is a misconception that Alzheimer's symptoms are part of the normal aging process. Although mild forgetfulness is common in people as they age, the worsening of memory decline, confusion, and other symptoms of Alzheimer's are due to the neurodegenerative nature of the illness. There are many people with mild cognitive impairment whose condition may not deteriorate to the extent to be diagnosed as Alzheimer's. However, there are others who will develop this illness, possibility due to genetic vulnerability or other reasons outlined in the risk-factor section of this book.[48]

Another misconception is that Alzheimer's disease does not cause death. This myth is probably derived from the observation that Alzheimer's patients may be able to live for ten to twenty years after diagnosis. Moreover, they usually have one or more other diseases, such as diabetes, hypertension, heart failure, or respiratory illness. These diseases can increase the risk of mortality before these patients reach the final stage of Alzheimer's. However, the physical and mental impact of neurological destruction of the brain eventually leads to death. In fact, Alzheimer's disease is listed as the sixth leading cause of mortality in the United States.[49]

Another myth is that Alzheimer's is caused by flu shots, aluminum, silver dental fillings, or aspartame (an artificial sweetener). None of these has been conclusively proven to be the case. Regarding any relationship between the flu shot and other vaccinations and Alzheimer's disease, in November 2001, the *Canadian Medical Journal* published a report that suggested that older adults who were vaccinated against diphtheria, tetanus, polio, or influenza seemed to be at lower risk of contracting Alzheimer's disease as compared with those who were not vaccinated. The notion of aluminum as a possible cause of Alzheimer's emerged in the 1960s and '70s. There was a concern about the use of or exposure to aluminum materials (e.g., pots, pans, and beverages cans). Research studies up to present have failed to show any evidence that aluminum causes Alzheimer's disease.[50]

Among other myths is the belief that Alzheimer's is a preventable disease that can be treated. Based on current scientific information, no effective and durable treatment to prevent, stop, or cure Alzheimer's disease has been found. There has been a great deal of publicity about what some believe to be cures or preventive treatments, including different diets, exercise, or herbal remedies and supplements; however, medical science has not yet discovered an effective treatment.[51]

Another misconception is that, through intellectual stimulation, the caregiver can help patients regain their lost memory. Consequently, in some families, the spouse or other caregivers may resort to harsh and relentless memory exercises whose results only create frustration and a feeling of helplessness in the patients. Although in the very early stage of Alzheimer's disease, some patients may benefit from certain intellectual exercises, unfortunately in the advanced stage, loss of memory will continue, and the ability to learn new intellectual skills or retrieve old memories will become increasingly impossible unless an effective and curative medication is found.

In their book, *The 36-Hour Day*, Mace and Rabins extensively discuss issues pertaining to caring for patients with Alzheimer's disease. They urge caregivers to avoid confrontation or argumentation as a means to raise patients' awareness or help them to understand certain points. Life should be made as easy and simple as possible, avoiding complicated messages and signals, because patients with Alzheimer's disease cannot follow these for proper actions. Decision making can become particularly difficult when there are many choices. In normal circumstances, decisions are made on the basis of facts; in Alzheimer's patients, memory fails to assimilate and process the facts, often leading to decisions that are irrelevant to current situations.

Another misconception arises from the fact that patients with Alzheimer's disease generally look healthy prior to their terminal stage. Because of this healthy appearance, caregivers and friends are at times reluctant to recognize or accept the tragic impairment taking place within the brain of the patient. They expect sufferers to perform as well intellectually and emotionally as they appear physically.

Finally, there is a misconception that Alzheimer's patients are unaware of what is going on around them and are oblivious to their illness. Therefore, because of this and the loss of memory, these patients do not suffer much from the impact of the illness. But close observation indicates that unless in the advanced stage, many of these patients do experience an intuitive awareness and painful realization of their intellectual impairment, which they often deny.

As the symptoms of memory loss and forgetfulness begin to penetrate, most Alzheimer's patients, particularly those who have higher education, are conscious of this cognitive decline, which is progressive. Many may try to conceal their symptoms. But as the condition worsens, they become increasingly anxious, depressed, frightened, and sometimes agitated, as they feel that they are helplessly drifting away in the darkness of forgetfulness and are unable to have any control over their increasing incapacity. On the other hand, there are other patients who appear to be resigned to and calmly accept their condition.

Warning Signs of Alzheimer's Disease

Becoming familiar with the early signs and symptoms of Alzheimer's disease will help individuals and family members recognize the potential appearance of this illness. However, it may not be easy to detect them. In fact, those whose symptoms are evident today may have begun to develop the disease 5-15 or more years earlier. Its progress can be very slow and insidious. On the other hand, in those who protract the disease at a younger age, as mentioned above, the illness may advance faster and its impact may be greater. Approximately 5–10 percent of people develop Alzheimer's disease before age sixty-five. This is called early-onset Alzheimer's.

Significant efforts have been made through neuropsychological testing and, more recently, through MRI, computerized tomography (CT), and other brain-imaging tests to detect the development of Alzheimer's disease. Although it is not the purpose of this book to elaborate on the details of diagnostic features of this disease, a brief outline of potential warning signs of Alzheimer's, which has been developed by the Alzheimer Society of Canada, is printed here with their permission.[52]

10 Warning Signs

1. **Memory loss that affects day-to-day function**
   It's normal to forget things occasionally and remember them later: things like appointments, colleagues' names or a friend's phone number. A person with Alzheimer's disease may forget things more often and not remember them later, especially things that have happened more recently.
2. **Difficulty performing familiar tasks**
   Busy people can be so distracted from time to time that they may leave the carrots on the stove and only remember to serve them at the end of a meal. A person with Alzheimer's disease may have trouble with tasks that have been familiar to them all their lives, such as preparing a meal.
3. **Problems with language**
   Everyone has trouble finding the right word sometimes, but a person with Alzheimer's disease may forget simple words or substitute words, making her sentences difficult to understand.
4. **Disorientation of time and place**
   It's normal to forget the day of the week or your destination—for a moment. But a person with Alzheimer's disease can become lost on their own street, not knowing how they got there or how to get home.
5. **Poor or decreased judgment**
   People may sometimes put off going to a doctor if they have an infection, but eventually seek medical attention. A person with Alzheimer's disease may have decreased judgment, for example not recognizing a medical problem that needs attention or wearing heavy clothing on a hot day.

6. **Problems with abstract thinking**
   From time to time, people may have difficulty with tasks that require abstract thinking, such as balancing a cheque book. Someone with Alzheimer's disease may have significant difficulties with such tasks, for example not recognizing what the numbers in the cheque book mean.
7. **Misplacing things**
   Anyone can temporarily misplace a wallet or keys. A person with Alzheimer's disease may put things in inappropriate places: an iron in the freezer or a wristwatch in the sugar bowl.
8. **Changes in mood and behaviour**
   Everyone becomes sad or moody from time to time. Someone with Alzheimer's disease can exhibit varied mood swings—from calm to tears to anger—for no apparent reason.
9. **Changes in personality**
   People's personalities can change somewhat with age. But a person with Alzheimer's disease can become confused, suspicious or withdrawn. Changes may also include apathy, fearfulness or acting out of character.
10. **Loss of initiative**
    It's normal to tire of housework, business activities or social obligations, but most people regain their initiative. A person with Alzheimer's disease may become very passive, and require cues and prompting to become involved.

Risk Factors

Although the cause of Alzheimer's disease is not known, there are a number of factors that predispose individuals to this disease. Age is the most important risk factor of Alzheimer's disease, but this disease is not part of the normal evolution of aging. Another factor is genetic disposition and family history. It is estimated that approximately 5–7 percent of Alzheimer's disease cases can be accounted for by inherited genes. In their review article, Xu, Ferrari, and Wang indicate that if one has a first-degree relative, such as a parent, brother or sister, with Alzheimer's disease, one is more likely to develop this disease as compared with those who don't have a first degree relative with Alzheimer's. Likewise, if there is more than one such relative, the risk is higher to develop the disease.[53] It is to be noted that, as mentioned above, there are environmental and other factors that can also influence the development of Alzheimer's.

Gender also plays a role. The prevalence of Alzheimer's disease is reported to be higher in women than in men. This may be partly due to the fact that women live longer than men and also because of environmental influences and hormonal changes in women.[54] Furthermore, seven potentially modifiable risk factors for this disease have been identified: diabetes, midlife hypertension, midlife obesity, smoking, depression, cognitive inactivity or low education achievement, and physical inactivity. [55]

It is to be kept in mind that Alzheimer's disease is influenced by all the above factors and their interactions. Research projects that are population based and prospective studies are more likely to identify factors that would influence the lifetime occurrence of dementia, including Alzheimer's. As mentioned before, age is one of the most powerful factors in the development of Alzheimer's disease. Increasing age also affects the role of different risk and protective factors during one's life-span.

Medical Diseases as Possible Risk Factors

There are a number of medical diseases that researchers have identified as potential risk factors for Alzheimer's disease:

Cardiovascular diseases and diseases of blood circulation: There are several cardiovascular disorders that may contribute to the development of Alzheimer's. High blood pressure in midlife may increase the risk of dementia and Alzheimer's, especially if high blood pressure has been a long-term problem. Interestingly when people get much older (over eighty) the effect of high blood pressure will be less, whereas low blood pressure may lead to the occurrence of dementia and Alzheimer's disease (probably because, as a result of low blood pressure, less blood reaches the brain cells). Thus, a normal blood flow and healthy blood circulation is important for brain functioning.

Cardiovascular disease, including heart failure, is associated with a higher risk of Alzheimer's disease. Moreover, an impediment in natural blood circulation may increase the risk of dementia, including Alzheimer's. For example, cerebrovascular disorders, such a stroke due to brain hemorrhage (infarct) and an ischemic condition of the cortical and other parts of the brain, may increase the likelihood of the incidence of dementia.[56]

Researchers at the University of California–San Francisco (UCSF) completed a longitudinal study of approximately thirty-five hundred adults to determine if there is any relationship between exposure to cardiovascular risk factors—that is, adverse lifestyle behaviors in early adulthood (ages eighteen to thirty) and cognitive decline during midlife (age forty-three to fifty-five). Adverse lifestyle behaviors include physical inactivity, poor diet, and so on. The study lasted for twenty-five years. The results showed that some of the risk factors, such as elevated blood pressure and low physical activity during the period of the study, were associated with worse cognitive performance during the midlife period.

According to Kristin Yaffe at UCSF, these research findings are critical in identifying the antecedents of diseases related to aging, such as cognitive impairments, years before the diagnosis of these conditions (e.g., dementia) is made. Such identification will provide an opportunity for intervention and prevention. Likewise, treatment of hypertension or other cardiovascular diseases may reduce the chance of developing cognitive impairment as mentioned in this book.[57]

Diabetes: The association of diabetes and cognitive impairment has been known in medicine for decades. Some reports suggest that type 2 diabetes is linked to cognitive decline, including memory impairment. It is believed that midlife diabetes or diabetes of long duration may play a critical role in the development of dementia and Alzheimer's. In general, diabetes is associated with a decrease in cognitive performance and a high risk for dementia.[58]

Obesity: In the research literature, lifetime obesity is also linked to an increased risk for dementia. Obesity during middle age may predispose an individual to dementia in later life, when the body weight may decrease to a normal or lower than normal weight.[59]

Benzodiazepines and Alzheimer's disease: Recent research findings suggest a potential link between benzodiazepines, a group of prescription tranquilizers, and the development of Alzheimer's. According to an article published in the *Journal of the American Medical Association* (*JAMA*) in December 2014, "Benzodiazepines are one of the most commonly prescribed psychotropic medications in developed countries."[60] The authors of this article indicate that the use of benzodiazepine by older individuals poses serious adverse effects, such as the impairment of cognitive function and driving skills, reduced mobility, and increased risks of falls.

According to recent reports from the National Institutes of Health (NIH) in the United States, "These medications [benzodiazepines] can pose real risks and there are often safer alternatives available."[61] The NIH expressed its concern over the fact that "prescription use of benzodiazepines increases steadily with age, despite the known risks for older people."[62] Another study reported in the *British Medical Journal* found that the association between the use of benzodiazepines and Alzheimer's was stronger if the medication was taken for a longer period of time.[63]

NIH further reported that, based on a study, "In all age groups, women were about twice as likely as men to receive benzodiazepines. Among women aged sixty-five–eighty years, 1 in 10 was prescribed one of these medications, with almost a third of those receiving long-term prescriptions."[64] In view of the above research data, the NIH stated that the pattern of prescribing benzodiazepines for older people and especially women was worrisome.

As these research findings on benzodiazepines are emerging, readers are advised to discuss the advisability of their use with their physicians. This group of medications is usually prescribed for the treatment of sleep disorders and anxiety and, like any other medications, have benefits and side effects. Therefore, before any change, consult with your doctor.

Sleep and Alzheimer's: According to the American Academy of Neurology, research reports suggest a possible relationship between sleep difficulties and vulnerability to dementia. A recent study suggests that sleep deprivation or disturbance may raise the level of amyloid deposition in the regions of the brain, which are affected in Alzheimer's disease. There have been a few other reports on the matter. According to Bryce Mander from the University of California–Berkeley, "Sleep appears to be a missing piece in the Alzheimer's puzzle, and enhancing sleep may lessen the cognitive burden that Alzheimer's disease impacts."[65] These hypotheses, however, need further exploration. It remains to be seen whether sleep disturbance increases amyloid deposition in the brain or if the opposite may also be true—that neurodegeneration of the brain produces disturbances in sleep.[66] There is a possibility that insufficient deep sleep may impact memory function in the long term. But none of the above and other findings have been clearly confirmed by science.[67]

Cigarette smoking and alcoholism: The relationship between tobacco smoking and cognitive impairment has been debated. Whereas some research reports suggest that there is an increased risk for Alzheimer's disease among smokers, other findings don't support this. Although in general, there seem to be more data in favor of the association of smoking and Alzheimer's, more research studies are needed to clarify this relationship.[68]

Consumption of excessive alcohol may lead to alcoholic dementia. There are indications that those who are involved in heavy alcohol intake during their middle-age years are more prone to increased risk of dementia in later age.[69]

There have also been studies on the role of other factors as possible contributors to the development of Alzheimer's disease, including lifestyle, diet and nutrition, education level, economic status, depression, head trauma, brain injury, occupational situations (i.e., exposure to electromagnetic fields), inflammation, and others.

Although medical science has yet to make significant progress in finding the most effective ways to prevent and cure Alzheimer's disease, by leading a healthier life with proper nutrition, physical and mental exercise, avoiding smoking and the other elements of potential high risk for this disease mentioned above, we may diminish the possibility of its development.

Protective Factors against Alzheimer's Disease

In contrast to risk factors, there are some emerging positive elements with possibly reducing or delaying effect on the development of Alzheimer's disease and probably other dementias. In light of the fact that the cause of Alzheimer's is not known, and there is no definitive treatment or cure for this illness, the following elements have been suggested in the literature to be beneficial. Some of these ideas have not been tested and proven for their effectiveness in spite of their popularity through the media. In fact, finding real "protective" or "preventive" factors is hard to come by, but efforts to break down the barriers to understanding how to delay or prevent dementia are potentially helpful.

Regular Exercise and Nutrition

Can regular physical exercise, diet, or lifestyle reduce the risk of developing Alzheimer's disease? How does it work, and what is the scientific evidence? There are indications based on scientific studies and behavioral observation to suggest that increased physical exercise and activities may prevent or delay the onset of dementia. It has been reported that physical activity during middle age can have a strong protective effect against the development of dementia and Alzheimer's disease in later life. However, such intense physical activity should continue, as it will take years until results are seen.[70]

Generally, people who engage in regular exercise or follow a healthy diet are those who are conscious of their physical well-being. On the other hand, our brain cells have a limited life-span, due to our human condition. Although we are able to prolong life with modern medical advancement and technology, we cannot turn back our biological clocks and regenerate new sets of brain cells or transform the cells and organs of our bodies into those of young people.

There has been increasing interest in the possible role of physical exercise in reducing the risk of or preventing Alzheimer's disease and consequent memory loss. In one study, changes in brain activity in older adults were explored with the use of MRI. Evaluation was done before and after a six-month program of brisk walking. Results indicated that activity of specific regions of the brain had increased. This may reflect a biological basis for the role of aerobic exercise, which would have possible beneficial effects on the cognitive function of older adults.[71]

A growing number of articles have been published in the medical literature during recent years containing commentaries and research findings about the significance of exercise, healthy food consumption, and improved lifestyle in efforts to prevent or delay cognitive impairment and dementia. Some of these publications are for the general public who may be interested to gain some insights.[72]

Can diet shield the aging brain?

A healthier diet has been hailed as another possible protective factor against the deterioration of brain function associated with aging. In a recent study, it was reported that a healthier diet in older adults can reduce impaired "executive function" of the brain by 35 percent. Executive function includes a number of important functions of the brain, such as memory, reasoning, planning, multitasking, and problem solving.[73]

Epidemiological studies have shown that foods rich in antioxidants like brightly colored fruits and dark-green, leafy vegetables may have a beneficial effect in preserving cognitive function. Likewise, antioxidants, by slowing the oxidation of other molecules, may reduce cell damage in the body. The effect of food rich in antioxidants was explored by a team of researchers at Harvard Medical School on thirteen thousand women aged seventy or older in the Nurses' Health Study.[74] This epidemiological study suggested that women who reported consumption of the largest amount of green, leafy vegetables (e.g., spinach, kale, and romaine lettuce) and cruciferous vegetables (e.g., broccoli, cabbage, brussels sprouts, and cauliflower) experienced lower levels of cognitive decline as compared with women who reported consuming smaller amounts of these vegetables.

Another epidemiological study of adults favored a "Mediterranean diet," which includes foods with nutrients rich in antioxidants and polyunsaturated fatty acids (PUFAs), such as fruits, vegetables, and fish; low to moderate quantities of dairy; fish; poultry; and frequent use of olive oil. It is suggested that this diet reduced the risk of Alzheimer's disease while prolonging the survival of people who suffered from this disease.[75] On the other hand, moderate to high intake of saturated fats may increase the risk of dementia and Alzheimer's disease. Fatty acids increase atherosclerosis and inflammation and, consequently, may enhance dementia.[76] In addition, a deficiency of B_{12} and folate (folic acid) have been noted to increase the possible risk of Alzheimer's disease. Recent research has shown that vitamin B supplements can help slow mental decline in older people with mild memory impairment if omega-3 fatty acid levels in their body are sufficiently high; however, more research is required in this area.[77]

There have been other studies that suggest beneficial effects of certain nutrients. Briefly, some researchers have found that cumin, which is an ingredient of curry and contains strong antioxidant and anti-inflammatory properties, may have preventive benefits for Alzheimer's disease. Other researchers have found that omega-3 fatty acid from fish reduces beta-amyloid and plaque levels in the brain.[78]

Among herbal remedies, the most popular is gingko biloba, which has been touted for its potential to improve memory in old age. Although this was noted to be true in some studies, most research findings have failed to prove its efficacy. A study carried out on over three thousand volunteers aged seventy and older showed that gingko did not provide any memory-preserving benefit, nor was it able to stop the progression of Alzheimer's. The results, published in the *Journal of Lancet Neurology*, were consistent with other previous findings.[79] Gingko, on the other hand, is a powerful antioxidant and also interacts with other medications. Therefore, those taking it with other medications should keep their doctors informed.

Coffee has been known for its stimulating effect on the brain. Researchers have reported that the consumption of caffeine/coffee is associated with a reduced risk of dementia or may delay its onset. Although the results of research studies on the positive effects of coffee in countering cognitive decline have been inconsistent, there are some studies to suggest that moderate drinking of coffee (three to five cups a day) during the midlife period will probably have a protective effect in decreasing the risk of developing dementia and Alzheimer's disease. While this and similar reports are intriguing, more vigorous research exploration is needed to confirm a relationship between drinking coffee and a delay or prevention of Alzheimer's disease and other dementia. The role of tea drinking on cognitive deterioration is less apparent. The mechanism of coffee intake in relation to dementia is not clear but may be due to its antioxidant and other effects yet to be explored.[80]

Mental and Physical Exercises

According to Norman Doidge, education and exercise, whether physical or mental, play important roles in rejuvenating the brain.[81] It has been reported that mental and physical exercises improve human brain function. However, not all activities have the same effect. Those activities that require concentration, like studying a musical instruction, reading, playing board games, and dancing, may lower the risk of Alzheimer's. Dancing requires much physical and mental concentration to learn new movements, and this is challenging for the mind. Doidge further comments that although these suggested activities may be helpful, they have not been proven to prevent Alzheimer's. "These activities are associated or correlated with less Alzheimer's, but correlations do not prove causality."[82]

Physical exercise is broadly useful in preserving well-being and preventing a number of medical illnesses. As the cause of Alzheimer's is not known, however, the effect of physical exercise should be viewed in the light of its correlation with lower risk for this disease. Physical exercise not only stimulates the body's defense against illness but also is likely to increase the production of new neurons and improve circulation, resulting in greater availability of oxygen for the brain. For example, physical exercises such as walking, cycling, and hiking strengthen the heart and blood vessels, including those in the brain, alleviate emotional tension, and sharpen the mind.[83]

Recent studies suggest that vigorous regular physical exercise will benefit the aging brain and may act as a buffer against symptoms of early Alzheimer's disease. It can also improve mood and memory. For example, it has been reported that aerobic exercise can improve blood circulation in key areas of the brain. It may also reduce the protein tangles in the brain caused by Alzheimer's disease.[84]

With aging, blood flow to the key areas of the brain decreases. Therefore, with a change of lifestyle and with more vigorous and regular aerobic exercise, this deficiency can be ameliorated, leading to better results, such as improved memory and attention.[85] However, more research is needed to substantiate this.

Psychosocial Protective Factors

Among psychosocial factors, the following are to be considered: educational achievement, mental stimulation, and socioeconomic status.

Education: According to Eric Kandel, "Learning leads to strengthening of synaptic connections."[86] Synapses between brain cells play an important role in transmitting information and facilitating the learning process. Wilder Penfield of McGill University was one of the pioneers in recognizing the storage of memory in the brain. While he was working on the brains of injured patients, he discovered that when he stimulated the medial temporal lobe of the brain and hippocampus, his patients reacted with hallucinations, or they remembered some experiences of the past.[87] Such findings underscore the role of education as a positive factor in preventing or delaying Alzheimer's.

Research studies have consistently shown that higher educational achievement in early life is associated with a lower incidence of dementia and Alzheimer's disease. Based on the cognitive-reserve hypothesis, childhood education probably enhances cognitive reserves, which provide "compensatory mechanisms to cope with degenerative pathology changes in the brain, and therefore delay onset of the dementia syndrome."[88] But there are exceptions to this, as there have been individuals, highly educated in the art and sciences, who developed Alzheimer's despite high educational achievement earlier in their lives. This factor supports the multifactorial nature of Alzheimer's disease and its causes.

If it is the case that higher education may serve as a protective factor to ward off dementia and Alzheimer's, what are the possible reasons for this development? Kenneth Langa and associates from the University of Michigan suggested the following as a probable explanation.[89] It is possible that schooling has a positive effect on brain development and that well-educated individuals may be more likely to undertake more cognitively demanding occupations as compared with less educated people. The greater demand on the brain might be a factor in warding off Alzheimer's disease. Another possibility is that "the brains of the better-educated individuals are able to sustain greater damage from Alzheimer's pathology…before reaching a threshold of clinical significance."[90] Alternatively, better-educated individuals may have a healthier lifestyle, controlling risk factors such as cardiovascular disorder, which might be detrimental to brain function. They also might have better access to the health care system and early intervention.

Cognitive stimulation: Besides the role of education as a contributing protective factor, early life experiences and cognitive stimulation are also important elements in the development of Alzheimer's. For example, crossword puzzles and other brain-stimulating games to enhance the mind are increasingly used to help keep the maturing brain sharp. The earlier such stimulating activities begin and the longer they are continued, the better it is.

A research study conducted on religious orders (including older nuns, priests, and religious brothers) who were followed for four years found that information-processing activities were associated with higher cognitive activity and reduced risk of developing Alzheimer's disease.[91] However, such findings must be taken with caution. One might even wonder if these activities have any relevance to the etiology of Alzheimer's, since the cause of it is still unknown. Moreover, a follow up survey of four or five years' duration is too short to determine a decreased or increased risk for Alzheimer's, as the disease can take one or two decades to develop.

There have also been observations and studies to suggest that people with higher socioeconomic status show decreased risk for developing

Alzheimer's disease. It is possible that most of those individuals had greater occupational opportunities because of their higher education.[92] But what about those in some parts of the world with very basic education who were able to achieve a high socioeconomic status? Are wealth and status a means of preventing Alzheimer's disease? Is it true that most Alzheimer's patients come from poor and uneducated populations? What about the role of cultural attitude and beliefs and also the effect of spiritual values and religious practices in curtailing the development of Alzheimer's disease? (Please see the section "Spiritual Dimensions" in this book.) These questions are raised to encourage reflection and to underline the need for more exploration.

Isolation as a risk factor: Isolation and limited social interactions and engagement in later life have been reported to be associated with an elevated risk of dementia. This may partly explain why there is a spike in the incidence of Alzheimer's disease after the age of retirement (in most parts of the world, around age sixty to sixty-five) and another jump around age eighty to eighty-five. The latter is probably a period of life when aged people (especially women) lose their spouses, their children have established their independent individual or family lives, and many former colleagues or friends have moved or passed away, and because of retirement, they have less active interaction with others; thus, social networking is poor. In addition, they are more likely to be affected by medical illness, which further limits mobility and social engagement. By this age, there is greater prevalence of inflammatory disease, diabetes, high blood pressure, cardiac disease, stroke, and so on, all of which increase the risk for dementia. Isolation and withdrawal may also be the consequence of dementia and not necessarily a factor leading to dementia.

Researchers have noted that involvement in complex social networks that enhance constant engagement and interaction with others has a beneficial effect on the brain. One research report points out that "people with complex social networks are constantly engaging with others in this way, updating their brain files. Perhaps, like formal education, this stimulates the brain and creates more cognitive reserve."[93] Hence, engaging in social activity and having many friends with whom one has frequent discussions and conversations seems to be associated with less cognitive deficit and lower risk of dementia in older age.

Despite the above research reports, the real connection between education, cognitive stimulation, social engagement, and Alzheimer's disease requires more investigation. It is not certain that mental stimulation as a means of intervention can exert a definite positive impact on the risk of developing Alzheimer's disease. In brief, educational activities, social interaction, and cognitive stimulation are positive and helpful activities for a healthy life, but whether they have a potential influence on the prevention of Alzheimer's disease requires more vigorous scientific research for a better understanding of their effect on cognition.

Finally, the good news is that, in contrast to public perception, a large number of elderly people with cognitive impairment are not affected by dementia. According to an American study, it was estimated that 22 percent of people aged seventy or over had cognitive impairment without dementia, and in Europe, studies reported the same phenomenon, with a prevalence of 21–27 percent among elderly people.[94] In many of these populations under study, the cognitive impairment was mild. This again further underlines the multifactorial nature of Alzheimer's disease and the interaction between biological and environmental forces.

Memory Changes

In a survey published in 2015, it was reported that within as many as one in eight households in the United States, there may be an adult with worsening memory loss or confusion. In an additional survey, it was noted that almost half of adults aged forty-five years or older have experienced memory loss or confusion and have admitted that these cognitive problems interfere with their daily life.

Both studies were conducted by US Centers for Disease Control and Prevention (CDC). The first study consisted of a telephone survey of over eighty-one thousand households in thirteen states. In each household, an adult member was asked whether any adult person in the home was experiencing memory loss or confusion that had worsened or become more frequent during the past twelve months. The data of the second survey mentioned above indicated that those who were the youngest in the age group (those closer to forty-five years old) were the most likely to report a memory problem.[95]

It is to be noted that the results of a telephone survey cannot be interpreted as a medical diagnosis. However, it is important to recognize that these early symptoms of memory problems may be a warning sign and require intervention before it is too late.

Aging and Memory Changes

As we age, the external signs of aging, such as graying hair, wrinkles and other skin changes, reduced eyesight, difficulty in hearing, diminished physical reflexes, and so on, appear. There are also internal physical changes that are associated with the wear and tear of aging as well as disturbances due to illnesses. These affect the muscles, bones, lungs, heart, and brain. Cognitive and memory decline are normal processes that are experienced as the brain ages. However, the destruction of brain cells brought on by dementia, including Alzheimer's, is a neurological disease, with emotional and intellectual deterioration, which also affects daily life and behavior.

The aging brain goes through structural changes, including loss of brain cells and atrophy of the brain, which could be mild or, in the case of Alzheimer's and other diseases, extensive. Some parts of the brain, such as the frontal and temporal lobes, are more affected by atrophy than other parts. The frontal lobes play an important role in the strategic application of memory and systematic memory search, which includes executive functions. The temporal lobes, which also include the hippocampus, serve to associate and retrieve information acquired in life.[96]

Besides these changes in the anatomy of the brain, there are also changes in its chemical structure, more specifically in the role of certain neurotransmitters such as acetylcholine and dopamine. These two neurotransmitters are important for communication between brain cells, or neurons. A neurotransmitter is a chemical substance that transmits nerve impulses across a synapse. With aging, the activity of these neurotransmitters will decrease in the brain.[97]

There is a notion that the cognitive changes of the natural aging process and severe cognitive deterioration of dementia are two extremes along a continuum of brain functioning in old age. However, this concept might lead one to perceive Alzheimer's or other dementias as a possible outcome of the normal process of aging and not as destructive diseases affecting the brain. It might also imply that the mild cognitive decline of aging will always progress to a form of dementia; however, this is not the case. In fact, "Mild cognitive impairment does not necessarily lead to dementia, but dementia is preceded by mild cognitive impairment and normal aging."[98]

Although progressive memory impairment is a characteristic symptom of Alzheimer's disease, a distinction should be made between abnormal memory loss and normal forgetfulness. The following table shows some features of normal and abnormal memory loss.

Changes in normal memory during aging may not, at times, be easily differentiated from mild cognitive impairment. Researchers (Anderson et al. 2012) believe that the most common memory challenge that appears as we age is remembering the names of new acquaintances and even those of people we have known for a very long time especially if we unexpectedly meet them in a context other than the one to which we are accustomed. Other memory mistakes commonly occur when we are not paying attention to a task at hand—for example, not remembering where we put our keys or glasses because we were probably not paying attention or were distracted when we put the item down. Such challenges are part of normal aging. As is indicated in the table below, an older person who forgets something and who is not affected by dementia will remember later, as compared with a patient with dementia who will not recall what he or she has forgotten.

Average Person	Alzheimer's Patient	Older Person
Is seldom forgetful	Often forgets entire experiences (e.g., may not remember eating and demands a meal)	Forgets part of an experience (e.g., can remember eating but doesn't remembers what fruit was served at lunch)
Remembers later	Rarely remembers later	Often remembers later
Acknowledges memory lapses lightly	Acknowledges lapses grudgingly after initial denial and attempts to compensate for lapse	Acknowledges lapses readily, often with a request for help in recalling information
Maintains skills, such as reading words or music	Skills deteriorate	Skills usually remain intact
Follows written or spoken directions easily	Increasingly unable to follow directions	Usually able to follow directions
Can use notes or reminders	Increasingly unable to use notes or reminders	Usually able to use notes or reminders
Can care for self	Increasingly unable to care for self	Usually able to care for self

Reprinted with permission of the American Psychiatric Association, 1992 [99]

In differentiating normal age-related memory decline from mild cognitive impairment (MCI) it is important to note that in MCI, there is subjective awareness of memory loss as well as objective memory impairment (measured by means of special testing). However, in MCI, there is no sign of generalized cognitive impairment or any symptoms of dementia, such as changes in behavior, character, and cognitive functioning, which one would find in cases of Alzheimer's.[100] On the other hand, MCI could develop into Alzheimer's as a person ages, especially if there is a genetic and family history of the disease.

Although memory impairment is a common symptom of Alzheimer's disease, as the condition progresses, other cognitive and behavioral symptoms will appear. Difficulty in remembering recent events while being able to recall events that occurred long ago is believed to be due to the inability to transform information arising in the short term into long-term memory. This process is called consolidation. With the progress of the disease, the long-term memory also gradually deteriorates. Getting lost in familiar places is also the result of an inability to remember these places as well as a disruption in spatial processing.

Anderson et al. noted that "memory processes include getting information into your memory (*encoding*), holding onto it over time (*storage* or *retention*), and getting it back out when you need it (*retrieval*). Normal aging has different effects on these memory processes. There is little effect of normal aging on the process of storage. At any age, as time goes by since you learned something new, you are less likely to remember it."[101] The above authors further observed that with normal aging comes a slight decline in encoding, making it a little more difficult. This challenge becomes much more common in older people. Difficulty in remembering a name is one of the most frequent memory complaints, and this is due to the failure of memory retrieval. It is to be noted that encodement, storage, and retrieval are interrelated processes.[102]

Creativity and Dementia: A Silver Lining

THE HUMAN BRAIN is an amazing organ with an extremely complex and well-organized network of communication signals between nerve cells. This center of the nervous system is composed of over one hundred billion nerve cells (neurons), which are interconnected. There are more than one hundred trillion connections at work in the human brain. In dementia, including Alzheimer's disease, although cognitive disturbances and decline, including forgetfulness, prevail, and a patient's language and daily behavior are adversely affected, scientists have discovered a silver lining of hope, which, in the past, was not recognized or not reported. That discovery is the appearance of certain artistic interests and activities, in some cases without any precedent in the life of these individuals. In some other cases, the artistic ability of patients continued unabated in spite of Alzheimer's disease. A report by researchers shows that in the case of a particular Alzheimer's patient, artistic productivity continued unaffected while he was suffering from progressive mental deterioration. This observation was interpreted by the researchers as a sign of resilience of human creativity, even in a case of dementia.[103]

Several researchers have indicated that although dementia is known to be associated with cognitive deficit, some previously acquired artistic skills and talents may be preserved in spite of the appearance of this degenerative disease. Some patients with dementia were reported to have maintained musical skills, ability in painting, and the capacity to engage in word games. [104, 105]

A case in point was a sixty-eight-year-old man with a twelve-year history of dementia. Previously, he had no interest in art and was a businessman. At age fifty-six, when his dementia began, he started to paint images. By age fifty-eight, his cognitive function, language, and memory had deteriorated. However, in spite of these changes, he was able to produce paintings with heightened precision and detail during the following years. More surprisingly, between the ages of sixty-three and sixty-six, his paintings won awards at art shows. He was evaluated at age sixty-eight, and it was noted that he had reduced facial emotions but heightened awareness of his environment. His MRI test showed a bitemporal atrophy of the brain.[106]

Emergence of Musical Abilities in Demented Patients

Literature on the role of music and music therapy in patients with dementia suggests that music/music therapy can serve as an effective intervention to improve dementia patients' social, emotional, and cognitive skills. Proper kinds of music are also reported to be helpful in reducing patients' behavioral problems. However, the mechanism of the therapeutic effect of music on the brain is not clear.[107]

There have been other reports from the American Academy of Neurology that show that creative abilities of different kinds, such as musical ones, may surface during the development of cognitive decline in some patients who suffer from frontotemporal dementia. Neurologist Bruce Miller et al. conducted an interesting study of twelve patients suffering from frontotemporal dementia. The results showed that in spite of worsening of cognitive and verbal abilities, their musical and visual capabilities were maintained or enhanced.[108]

Among these patients was a forty-nine-year-old man without previous musical ability who developed a progressive kind of aphasia and dementia. He used to be gifted in foreign languages and had received a master's degree in linguistics. At age forty-two, he became withdrawn but would constantly whistle. He began to show musical ability and composed musical songs about his bird. In contrast to his previous shyness, he became inappropriately exuberant. At age forty-seven, he began to experience memory difficulties and was forced to retire. He was evaluated through neuropsychological tests that confirmed a subtype of dementia affecting the right temporal lobe of his brain.[109]

Singing indeed has been reported to possibly have a beneficial effect on brain function. A group of Finnish researchers conducted a study of eighty-nine individuals with mild to moderate dementia. The participants were followed for ten weeks, during which they were either coached in singing, given familiar songs to listen to, or received standard care from their caregivers. The study showed that those who were coached in singing demonstrated improved memory and thinking skills, especially if they were younger than eighty years old and had mild dementia. Among those who listened to music, beneficial effects were more evident in those who had more advanced dementia. Having previous musical experience, either through singing or playing a musical instrument, did not influence the beneficial effect of the music therapy experience of the study's participants. It is to be noted that the sample for this study was small, but nevertheless, the authors concluded that singing might be beneficial for Alzheimer's patients.[110]

There have also been reports regarding patients with a history of artistic ability, including painting and other visual arts, who developed dementia. Although they suffered cognitive decline and deterioration, some of them continued to show ability to create artwork of good quality.

However, it should not be generalized that all dementia or Alzheimer's patients will develop such abilities nor that they will be able to maintain the creative skills that they possessed prior to their developing dementia.

As to whether there are two separate brain centers responsible for two different phenomena of cognitive skills and performance versus artistic abilities requires more research exploration. What is very intriguing is that as part of the brain is damaged by a neurodegenerative disorder causing cognitive deterioration, another part of the brain is triggered to discharge artistic and musical impulses for unusual performance. Is this a form of compensation within the ailing brain among the aging population? Although there may not be an easy answer at present, this discovery of a silver lining in degenerative brain diseases such as dementia and Alzheimer's is very intriguing. Future scientific studies may illuminate the nature and mechanism of this paradox of destruction and creative expression in the life of a brain struck by dementia.[111]

Carlos Hugo Espinel proposed a term for the emergence of something positive and creative from a degenerative sickness like dementia. He called it "Creating in the Midst of Dementia."[112] Briefly, his concept of a combination of brain function and malfunction is related to a trigger for brain reactivation. This trigger would possibly bring about a "cognitive repair" and lead to creating in the midst of dementia. This hypothesis is interesting but needs to be further examined.

Treatment of Alzheimer's Disease

Research toward discovering a cure for this illness has been intensified in recent years. Despite significant progress, finding a cure has been as elusive as uncovering a cause. Alzheimer's disease is a complex illness characterized not only by impairment of intellectual function but also by behavioral and personality deterioration, making its treatment more complex. In recent years, the cholinergic theory of this illness has attracted considerable interest and has led to the discovery of medications, which, for the first time, have brought about symptomatic improvement of memory functioning in some patients, although it does not have a lasting and curative effect. This approach was based on observations suggesting loss of cholinergic neurons in some parts of the brain.

The role of cortical cholinergic dysfunction of the brain and the effect of cholinesterase are being investigated. Likewise, the influence of amyloid accumulation and the impact of vascular risk factors such as hypertension and high cholesterol are being explored in search of a remedy. These and many other scientific research studies may illuminate the path toward prevention and effective treatment of this disease.[113]

During the past thirty years, there has been significant scientific research focused on discovering an effective treatment for Alzheimer's disease and other dementias. But to date, none of the medications has proven to have a lasting effect in curbing the degenerative impact of

Alzheimer's disease. Most medications marketed for Alzheimer's belong to the group of central cholinesterase inhibitors. The choice of these medications in the treatment of Alzheimer's is based on the notion that they act by raising brain acetylcholine levels and increasing cholinergic brain activity.[114]

The first medication approved by the FDA (Federal Drug Administration) for the treatment of Alzheimer's disease was Tetrahydroaminoacridine (Tacrine), which was an old medication from Australia. Initial reports showed a very positive effect on Alzheimer's, but subsequent controlled research trials of Tacrine in dementia revealed that although it was useful with modest effect on mild to moderate cognitive impairments, it had a toxic effect on the liver and, therefore, unfortunately, could rarely be used.[115]

The next drug to be introduced, which has been commonly used up to present for treatment of Alzheimer's, is Donepezil (Aricept). It is a safer medication than Tacrine, but it is not more effective. It can modestly improve cognitive function and the quality of the life of patients and is well tolerated, except for its gastrointestinal and a few other side effects, which are dose related.

There have been a few other new medications that increase acetylcholine and exert therapeutic effect on the treatment of Alzheimer's disease. These include Rivastigmine (Excelon), Galantamine (Reminyl), and Memantine (Namenda). Memantine was the first medication approved for treatment of moderate to severe types of Alzheimer's disease. Its mechanism of efficacy is different than that of previous medications. It is efficacious, with better side-effect profile and has been well adapted in clinical practice. It can also be used in combination with some other cholinesterase inhibitors.[116] Although these medications, especially Donepezil, which has been much studied, and Memantine, which is viewed as an important addition, have mild to moderate effects, there is still a long way to go to find a medication that will successfully cure Alzheimer's disease.

Nevertheless, there is a range of scientific research studies that seek to unlock the mystery of successful treatment of this disease, which affects millions of people around the world and deprives them of the most cherished gift of lifetime memory and personal identity.

Nonpharmacological remedies such as herbs and nutritional supplements, from omega 3 to coconut oil and from ginkgo biloba to vitamins, have been widely publicized in the media and are acclaimed as boosters of memory. Although there have been reports of some cognitive improvements through the use of very few of these substances, their effectiveness in the treatment of Alzheimer's disease has not yet been proven through rigorous scientific research evidence. However, as mentioned in another part of this book, daily mental and physical exercise as well as attention to quality of nutrition; avoidance of smoking, inactivity, and obesity; and prevention of head injuries or stroke will be important (please also see the section on risk factors). In the light of the above, discovering an effective treatment for this neurodegenerative disease is a work in progress. Let's hope that it will not take too long.

Besides memory and cognitive problems, Alzheimer's patients also experience mood and behavioral symptoms as the illness progresses, as well as possible delusions and hallucinations. For these and other symptoms, careful evaluation is required to ensure proper pharmacological management. Among mood disorders, depression is frequently reported. In one report, approximately 40–50 percent of Alzheimer's patients felt depressed, while 10–20 percent of those suffered from depressive disorder that required treatment including antidepressants. In addition, some Alzheimer's patients may need attention and treatment for anxiety, agitation, insomnia, paranoia, and other emotional or physical symptoms.[117]

Research studies show music can have a positive effect on the memory and behavior of patients suffering from dementia including Alzheimer's. The role of music and music therapy in treating patients with psychiatric disorders as an adjunct therapy is not new. But its influence in stimulating memory in patients with Alzheimer's is an interesting development requiring more exploration. Does certain music unlock the mind and memory in patients who harbor a degenerative brain disorder? How does it work?

A review of twenty-one empirical studies involving 336 patients suffering from dementia showed encouraging results. It was reported that, overall, the effect of music/music therapy was significant.[118] However, although music may have a calming effect on the behavior of Alzheimer's patients or may stimulate memory, it should not, at present, be perceived as an effective treatment to prevent the fading of memory in these patients. It also depends on the type of music and the patient's past experience with it. Certain kinds of music may calm, while others may excite or agitate patients with dementia. I know of a bright Polish engineer who developed Alzheimer's disease in his seventies. It progressively worsened with loss of memory, confusion, disorientation, paranoid thoughts, and the need for constant care at a geriatric care facility. He gradually lost his ability to walk and talk, and he hardly recognized friends and family. Throughout his life, he had loved to listen to classical music. When his illness reached an advanced stage, despite his mental and physical impairment, he would instantly respond to classical music, as was evidenced by his facial expression and bodily movements. Recognition of a musical melody that he had enjoyed in the past was the last remnant of memory to which he could relate with joy, despite the loss of almost all other memories. This demonstrates that not all parts of his cognitive function and memory had disappeared. Thus, music does have some effect on Alzheimer's patients, especially music that was part of their personal and cultural experiences in the past.

Likewise, prayer may enhance serenity in those who were religious or spiritually oriented during their life before the onset of the disease. Reciting a prayer at the bedside of a patient may, at times, bring a sense of calmness and peace for a moment or longer. Does prayer always require intact cognitive ability in order to be effective or to be felt? How is it that a patient with a degenerative brain disease is able to experience something that is a nontangible and spiritual experience? Can spirituality transcend the physical impairment of the cognitive function of the brain? As the human spirit is a nonmaterial and metaphysical entity, science is unable to explain such experiences with its conventional tools and laboratories. There must be another dynamic human process at work that our current scientific system of knowledge is unable to unravel. It is said that prayer is a language of the soul, which may connect the caregiver with the patient.

Caring for Patients with Alzheimer's Disease

THE MOST FORMIDABLE challenge facing the family is to accept the reality of the illness—that it exists, that it has struck a friend or loved one, and that it will persist until the end of the patient's life unless medicine discovers a cure. Because there is no cure for Alzheimer's disease at present, long-term care for these patients is a major challenge for family members and other caregivers. Indeed, it has been reported that approximately one-third of those caring for patients with Alzheimer's disease suffer from exhaustion and stress as well as from injuries sustained as a result of the physical task of caring for these patients. [119]

In caring for patients with Alzheimer's disease or other forms of dementia, one should look beyond the person who is mentally afflicted and confused. According to 'Abdu'l-Bahá, "The mind is circumscribed, the soul is limitless. It is by the aid of such senses as those of sight, hearing, taste, smell and touch, that the mind comprehendeth, whereas, the soul is free from all agencies. The soul as thou observest, whether it be in sleep or waking, is in motion and ever active. Possibly it may, whilst in a dream, unravel an intricate problem, incapable of solution in the waking state."[120] Caregivers should reach for that limitless soul. As the patient becomes increasingly inaccessible through verbal communication, greater effort should be made to establish and maintain a contact with his or her feelings and spiritual capacity—his or her soul. But how do we know if we are in touch with the feelings of someone who cannot respond adequately to a question? How can we reach a person's soul when that person despises us as strangers, never to be trusted? This is a most difficult challenge, particularly in the Western world, where emphasis is more on the mind and intellect than on feeling and intuition. People don't know how to relate to one another through their soul, fearing that they may be accused of being superstitious. Spiritual contact through prayer and meditation and the unconditional love and affection shown by family and friends will facilitate the contact these patients can feel, a contact that becomes increasingly necessary when verbal communication becomes meaningless or impossible. If caregivers make a new adjustment to the needs of the patient, a new journey can begin.

Often family members and caregivers of an Alzheimer's patient are frustrated and concerned with the "mirror" and not the "sun." They don't look for the rays of the soul beyond the "mirror." They judge the patient according to their own values and find the result disappointing. Caregivers are like co-travelers of patients with Alzheimer's disease, who need accompaniment to complete their journey through this world with the help of their friends and loved ones. This journey is too difficult for the patient to bear all alone. The co-travelers, for their part, will discover new mysteries of the reality of this journey of life. Although it appears a very strenuous physical and mental journey, it is also a spiritual companionship. It is an act of faith more than an act of reason.

Some very moving and personal stories of caring for a family member afflicted by Alzheimer's disease come from caregivers who are adult children of such patients. The Alzheimer's Association has published on its website (www.alz.org) a number of these stories written by the caregivers themselves. A few of them are shared in this book with the Association's permission, one of which is as follows:

> My mother died five years ago, having suffered from Alzheimer's for about 10 years. It is usually not a clear moment when the illness strikes. As with many people, she was a healthy old woman, somewhat forgetful, a little absent minded, losing words here and there and forgetting names. It was a shock to me when she was officially diagnosed by the psychiatrist as suffering from dementia of the Alzheimer's type. More shocking for me, maybe, because I was working at the time, as an art therapist with Alzheimer's patients…
>
> It was very sad to witness the gradual deterioration, as parts of her were slowly lost to me and to the world. But I do want to mention something quite surprising. My mother was a woman with much talent, a love of art, and quite creative. However, she never really fulfilled her potential, always unsure of what she did and mostly devaluing her work and giving up without investing any real effort.
>
> However, an astonishing thing happened as her dementia progressed. She became less self-conscious, less self-critical and much more content with whatever creative work she was involved with. As an art therapist, I spent times with her, encouraging her to draw and paint. I would sit next to her, give her paper and different sorts of crayons and give her ideas of what to draw. I saw that she was easily satisfied with what she drew, even if it was not particularly impressive. "That's quite lovely," she would say, which she would never have done in the past. "I think I'd like to do another," she would continue. This was a strange contribution of the illness that gave her a certain freedom, as though

some internal critical voice was put to sleep and she could be who she was without putting herself down…

I know how many millions of people are seeking ways to help their parents or spouses or sisters or brothers who become more and more isolated by the illness. I know that art therapy does not cure the illness, but for many people, it increases quality of life, provides them with an "alternative" language, the language of art, through which to express emotions trapped inside.[121]

A large number of patients with dementia are being cared for and looked after by family members and relatives, who have their own share of pain and suffering. Caregivers receive little recognition or support for their never-ending hours of tedious responsibilities. Many of them silently sacrifice their comfort and freedom to go places, attend special events, visit friends and other relatives, have a break for a vacation, or even attend to other personal responsibilities. Caught between the moral duty to serve a helpless and dependent patient and the need to regain their energy, which has been drained from the stress of caregiving, they may become exhausted and distressed. Consequently, mixed feelings of anger and guilt may prevail, and these need to be recognized and addressed.

Alzheimer's disease and emotional intimacy: Generally, Alzheimer's disease is understood as a condition that largely affects memory and intellect. But as the disease progresses, emotional and sexual intimacy may be adversely affected for other reasons. For example, because of memory loss, a patient may perceive his wife as a stranger or imposter who is trying to invade his privacy and harm him. Sometimes, paranoid or other delusional ideas overcome his judgment, and he may become enraged toward his spouse, whom he perceives as an intruder. Obviously, this can be heartbreaking for his wife, especially if they were married for many years and raised children together.

The same can also happen if the wife suffers from Alzheimer's disease. For a similar reason of memory deficit and delusion, she may refuse to allow her husband to enter their home, accusing him of being a stranger or an imposter. Sometimes, men or women afflicted by Alzheimer's may identify a total stranger as a family friend or even one's spouse and seek emotional or sexual intimacy with that individual. Such behavior can cause outrage, anger, and resentment on the part of the real spouse, who, unaware of this irrational symptom of Alzheimer's disease, feels betrayed.

Alzheimer's disease does not necessarily diminish sexual feelings. In fact, it has been reported that sometimes individuals with Alzheimer's disease display hypersexuality or are overly interested in sexual intimacy. This can occur as another symptom of the disease and may not be rationally intended behavior.[122]

In a married couple where one spouse develops Alzheimer's, and the disease is progressing, usually sexual relations are not perceived as a priority because of the worries that affect family life, such as concern over debt, financial limitations or lack of resources, and the prospect of placement in a nursing home, to mention a few. But when the question of sexuality arises, couples may explore other nonsexual but intimate ways of spending time together. They may consider nonsexual forms of contact, such as hugging, touching, dancing, and making each other's presence felt. That way, the sexual needs become sublimated, and they assure one another of loving and caring for and accompanying one another. Also, it is possible that the lack of interest in a sexual relationship on the part of the Alzheimer's patient may be due to depression or the effects of the medications prescribed to remedy the symptoms of the illness.

Caring for a demented patient is a type of giving for which there is no return. There is little expression of gratitude or joy of acknowledgement from these patients to brighten the days of their caregivers. The attention span, judgment, and ability to recognize the loving care of others are too limited or impaired in the patient to allow him or her to express appreciation for the value of these services.

However, once in a while, there are glimmerings of love and recognition, as illustrated in the following account. The wife of an Alzheimer's patient who was tireless in caring for her husband despaired of ever being able to communicate with him. One day, as she was sitting next to him, he suddenly took her hand, looked into her eyes, and told her how much he appreciated her caring for him. These unexpected sweet words astonished her and brought tears to her eyes. Although shortly after, he slipped back into the shadows of Alzheimer's, she never forgot that moment. Glimmerings like these frequently occur before a patient descends into a more advanced stage of the illness when language becomes inaccessible. When they happen, such moments should be cherished.

Generally, on the other hand, caregivers tend to offer a great deal but see no improvement. When they express frustration about this situation, they need to be heard and understood. The following words of Bahá'u'lláh point out the great importance of their task: "Should anyone give you a choice between the opportunity to render a service to Me and a service to them [parents], chose ye to serve them, and let such a service be a path leading you to Me."[123]

Caring for Elderly Patients: A Family Affair

Before we begin to discuss the role of adult children or grandchildren in providing care for their parents or grandparents, let's briefly review the evolution of family life and parent-child relationships. Since the Industrial Revolution, there have been changes in the traditional extended family, which have led to the emergence of the nuclear family.[124] Although in some parts of the world, the extended family model still exists, in most industrialized countries, the nuclear family is prevalent. The separation of work and home has further affected intergenerational contact—in particular, contact with the elderly.

Because of the decrease in the birthrate, partly due to the nuclear family lifestyle and the large number of childless marriages, the number of grandchildren has decreased during the past twenty-five years, and this trend will continue in the future. This will have an impact on the availability of children and grandchildren to have close contact with and to care for their parents and grandparents.[125]

Due to a breakdown in the institution of marriage, an increase in the rate of separation and divorce, and the rise of common-law partnerships, the likelihood that grandparents will be able to spend time with their grandchildren has declined. In 2008, during a trip to northern China, I was invited to visit a hospital's geriatric department. I was surprised to see that in such a well-organized department, one could see hardly any visitors. During visiting hours, the elderly patients were virtually alone, except for nurses who were attending to them. Knowing that the Chinese culture lays great emphasis on the value and integrity of the family and respect for elderly parents and grandparents, I asked the nurse of that department why there were no visitors. She explained that, because of the one-child policy in China, the young adult children, who, after marriage, are very busy with their work and own family, have little time left for visiting. Moreover, the hospital was located a two-hour drive away from the city, which made it difficult for loved ones to visit. In view of the situation, the hospital had hired nursing assistants or attendants to visit and spend some time with those elderly patients whose children or grandchildren were unavailable to attend.

The above dilemma is sad, because in Chinese cultural tradition, especially in the rural areas and villages, the elderly have been valued and cared for by family members, including children, or by the community from which the children have moved in order to work in the cities. It seems that with the advent of modernization in mainland China, there are fewer elderly people in cities, partly because many return to their native villages when they grow older or are cared for in government facilities.

In spite of cultural variations among Asian peoples, large numbers of their population believe that old age is equated with an accumulation of wisdom and deserve more attention. Confucian concepts encourage filial piety and respect for parents, which is linked to the principle of the sanctity of ancestors. This sense of respect for the past and ancestor worship are associated with respect for parents. In brief, Asian societies value the unity of the family and respect for the role of elderly in society.[126] However, due to the influence of the materialistic perspective of the Western world, it remains to be seen how long these cultural values with regard to old people will remain intact.

Caring for an Alzheimer's patient has primarily been a family affair. If the person suffering from Alzheimer's disease is married, the spouse, regardless of gender, is most likely to act as the main caregiver. But if the Alzheimer's patient is widowed, this responsibility is often undertaken by an adult child. Depending on the family and cultural background, the individual who fulfils this role may vary. However, it is very likely to be a daughter or daughter-in-law.[127]

In most families, during the early stage of the illness, care is provided by members of the family rather than by formal support services or nursing homes, partly because of the heavy cost of support from the outside or for cultural or family reasons. However, later on, when the demented family member requires constant nursing or medical care, outside assistance becomes a pressing necessity.

Sometimes a few adult children of an Alzheimer's patient may develop a coordinated plan to work together as primary caregivers to look after a sick parent. The following is an insightful story of three sisters who combined their efforts to face this challenge.

> We made the group decision to help Mom get through this to the best of our abilities. I'm one of her daughters. Mom began showing signs of memory loss about 15 years ago at the age of 75 (then already a widow of seven years). There were subtle signs at first: repeated questions; confusion as to how to use the stovetop… repeated dialing of familiar phone numbers; and confusion as to how to apply her makeup. At that time, my two sisters and I took turns living with her and providing daily assistance. Back then we didn't "understand" dementia or Alzheimer's disease…
>
> When Mom lost her ability to walk at about the age of eighty-five, she became an official "stay at home" Mom. My two sisters and I changed our work schedules to accommodate Mom's needs for around the clock care. We found a couple of caregivers to assist with covering shifts when the three of us were not available. I moved in with my Mom…to provide her care and companionship in the evenings and help get her into bed each night, always with a wish for "sweet dreams." I truly miss those days; they were tender and sweet.
>
> My Mom passed just over a year ago, just shy of her 90th birthday…In her last earthly days, it was not Alzheimer's disease, but an acute lung infection that she struggled valiantly to overcome that took her last breath. We are blessed that in her last 48 hours of life, she was loved and comforted by her three daughters, attended to by her hospice nurse, and listened on the telephone to the voices of her two sons that lived out of state. I was honored to be with her at the last breath of her life; it was a sacred moment. She was beautiful, brilliant, a gifted writer, and the person I loved most on this earth.[128]

Alzheimer's is a daunting challenge for society. Dementia in general (and Alzheimer's in particular) constitutes one of the most critical public health problems among older people. Therefore, when the responsibility for care of such patients falls on the shoulders of an adult child, he or she should become well informed and be supported in order to be able to assume primary care of the elderly Alzheimer's patient. Some people perceive this responsibility as a challenge, because they were raised and loved by this elderly person who is now disabled. Others simply feel very close to the patient and see service as a primary caregiver as a blessing.

It is important to be mindful of the fact that adult children or grandchildren also have their hopes and dreams, such as completing their education, beginning a career, and marrying and having children. For some of those who are newly married, the task of being a caregiver plus adapting to a new stage in their own lives may be exacting, especially if they were not prepared for such a task or were forced to undertake this burden of responsibility. Such a situation may cause much stress and emotional difficulties. They may also feel isolated from their friends. On the other hand, the experience these young people gain through caring for their sick relatives may give them a better understanding of suffering and result in their developing great maturity through service to others.

In their study of 197 dementia patients aged sixty-five years or over in an urban-rural fringe area of China, Hong Li et al. (2012) explored the caring burden and associated factors of care providers for dementia patients. In that part of China, they reported, the prevalence rate of dementia was 7.3 percent. They found that the attitude of care providers toward their responsibility affected the level of burden they felt in their caring work. Their role awareness ranged from "being willing" to provide care and assume familial responsibility to feeling obligated to provide that care.[129] Those who considered their role in providing care as being an "obligation" scored higher in the physical toll this responsibility had on them as compared with care providers who felt "willing" to provide care."[130] The physical and emotional burden scores were also higher among care providers whose patients were physically disabled.

The above research finding underlines the significance of caregivers' attitude and the perception of the responsibility they undertake. "Willingness" reflects a greater intrinsic motivation on the part of the caregiver as opposed to "obligation," which may focus on to fulfilling a duty. However, sometimes it may be difficult to separate willingness from obligation. In concluding, Hong Li et al. noted the need for developing community care programs and services that would decrease the burden of family-based care providers.[131]

In caring for Alzheimer's patients, we should be aware of the needs of these patients, which are common to an aging population. Isolation and withdrawal are daily problems. This calls for companionship, which provides not only a sense of presence of a loved one or a caregiver but also a sense of security and assurance. Patients suffering from dementia, especially Alzheimer's, feel insecure and vulnerable because of progressive loss of mental functioning and ability to protect themselves. This insecurity feeds into their sense of mistrust and paranoid thinking.

Caregiving is a noble service that requires a lot of sacrifice, not only of time and energy but also of freedom. This being said, it will be important for caregivers to pay attention to their own health, emotional well-being, and achievement of personal goals and for those close to them to ensure that these needs are taken care of. Should this be neglected, the caregiver will often succumb to the effects of stress, which include angry and guilty feelings that may be overwhelming and lead to anxiety, depression, and a sense of failure. Family bonds and relationships may suffer, as discussed in the following section on caring for caregivers. Professional caregivers hired from outside (or volunteers who come in to give the family member a break) may not experience the same sense of personal obligation, as they can more easily detach themselves from their personal feelings and from the expectations of the family of the patient. However, in spite of the challenges that adult children of Alzheimer's patients may have to face, there are creative ways in which they can be overcome. The following is a case of an adult child of an Alzheimer's patient and her challenges:

> My mom was diagnosed with Alzheimer's disease five years ago. She's sixty now. It started shortly after my father died—there was depression, not eating, mild confusion and personal hygiene changes. We all believed she was just mourning the loss of my father.
>
> As her child, I saw more at first than the rest of my family: bounced checks, becoming lost, paranoia. Our worst fears were realized when we found out she had Alzheimer's. Not only had I just lost my father, but bit by bit I was losing my mother and my boys their grandmother.
>
> Three years ago, the neighbors found her wandering in her yard, claiming someone stole her pension check. I knew it was time to sell her house and ours, and to combine our families for whatever time she had left. She has declined greatly in the last few years. She's now in a diaper and talks to me as if I'm a child again. I believe that when she looks at me, she only sees the person who makes her shower and take her pills; who I really am to her is gone.
>
> My children are my champions; at only 12 and 13, they remind me every day why my mom is here and why I'm doing what I do. They know how bad it may get, but they have no fear—because she is Grandma. I don't dare tell them that I don't think she remembers their names. They know she loves them, and that's enough. For now, that's all we need; names may not be important, but love is, and it's there.[132]

Some research studies show that caring for a patient with dementia, although it provides a wonderful opportunity to care for someone, can also have a challenging impact on the mental, physical, and social aspects of the caregiver's life as well as on his or her career. However, these studies also suggest ways to improve coping skills to mitigate or prevent the negative consequences of caregiving. For example, they give advice on how to improve the efficacy of caregivers in their psychosocial interventions, taking into consideration the caregivers' interests as well as the state of illness of the sick parent. This applies to the mild to moderate stages of Alzheimer's, because as the condition further deteriorates, there will be a need for more professional and well-trained individuals to care for such patients. Nevertheless, by increasing one's knowledge about Alzheimer's disease and how to interact with patients, a more satisfactory relationship can develop between the caregiver and the patient. This would include a deeper understanding of the conceptual framework of caregiving, which enables the caregiver to attain a sense of confidence.[133]

Religious scriptures encourage people to honor their parents in recognition of their hardship in striving to raise and educate their children. Christ stated, "Honor your father and mother that it may go well with you, and that you may enjoy long life on the earth" (Eph. 6:2–3). In the Bahá'í writings, we find these emphatic words about children and their parents: "Rarely do the mother and father enjoy in this world the rewards of all the pain and trouble they have endured for their children."[134] Therefore, children are encouraged to compensate through charity, beneficence, and praying for their parents.

Sometimes when parents are sick and disabled (due to dementia or any other disabling disease), they feel that they are a burden on their children. They experience guilt in seeing their children having to sacrifice their time and rest to insure that they (the parents) are well taken care of and nursed. In a letter on behalf of Shoghi Effendi to a mother, these heartening words of advice are written: "Although in some ways you may be a…burden to your children, it is to them a privilege to look after you; you are their Mother and have given them life, and through the bounty of Bahá'u'lláh they are now attracted to His Faith. Anything they do for you is small recompense for all you have done for them."[135]

In the Bahá'í community, caring for elderly individuals (with or without dementia) has a special place. Bahá'í houses of worship in the future will have dependencies raised up around them for cultural and humanitarian activities and for the well-being of humanity. These dependencies will furthermore provide centers of education and scientific learning imbued with the spirit of service and worship to advance the social and spiritual progress of mankind.[136] Among these dependencies will be a center or facility for the care of elderly individuals. The significance of this arrangement is that individuals in their advanced age will enjoy calm, comforting, and spiritual surroundings as they prepare for their transition to the next world.

Caring Matters

Elderly patients need to be loved in addition to being cared for. Caregivers who cannot provide this praiseworthy quality of care with love and respect may not be able to provide compassionate care. There have been reports of abuse and mistreatment of patients in nursing homes or hospitals, which underlines the significance of being trained and prepared with qualities for this kind of task. On the other hand, caregivers also have their own needs, such as having time for themselves and overcoming the stress associated with caring for others. Nevertheless, patients are vulnerable as a result of the illness and depend on the assistance of caregivers.

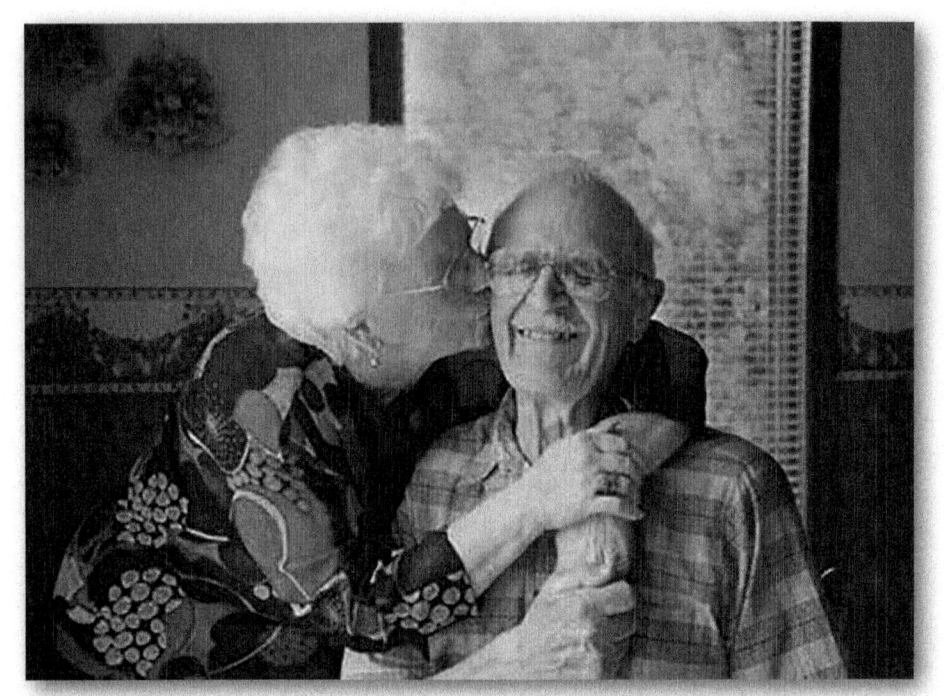

Copyright permission from Alzheimer's Disease International.[137]

Caring for Caregivers

As Alzheimer's is a serious and progressive disease and, based on current clinical knowledge, irreversible, it brings much pain and grief to family members. When caregivers face this discouraging and unalterable prognosis with respect to their loved ones, they may feel frustrated—a normal reaction. This feeling of frustration is at times compounded by a sense of despair and anger, directed not only toward the disease but also sometimes toward the patient, the doctor, and other resources as well as toward oneself for not being able to bring about a positive change in the patient. They may often feel guilty, thinking that they don't give enough. There are also feelings of loneliness and of being alienated from others—friends, colleagues, and other family members.

Caregivers are the "hidden victims"[138] of Alzheimer's disease who need a great deal of support and reassurance. Unfortunately, society has given them little attention or recognition. In reality, far from being inadequate, they give tirelessly of themselves, often succumbing to what is called "compassionate fatigue." In responding to a patient's needs, they overlook or deny their own needs, resulting in the feelings mentioned in the previous paragraph. Such sentiments should be acknowledged by others through showing tenderness and compassion toward caregivers and providing them with relief and comfort, since they are also human beings who are facing difficult and daunting tasks. The powerful emotions they feel need to be discussed and identified, and solutions need to be found to alleviate the situation. Caregivers may sometimes need counseling and therapeutic intervention themselves. If they become sick and unable to function, this will adversely affect the care of the patient who depends on the caregiver.

Today, in many parts of the world, there are local Alzheimer's societies or Alzheimer's associations, where family members and other caregivers can meet on a regular basis and share their own views and feelings. Through such periodic contact, they realize that they are not alone in their predicament and discover new ways of coping and caring for their loved ones. They need not only to be understood but also to be relieved from their burden of caring periodically so that they may attend to their own needs and regain their strength.

Coping with Caregiver Stress

Stress among caregivers of patients with dementia is a common and troubling problem. It has been reported that two-thirds of people who suffer from dementia live at home and are cared for by family members. Approximately 40 percent of family caregivers develop clinical symptoms of anxiety or depression. Eventually, these emotional problems lead to breakdown in care, and, as a result, those suffering from dementia need to be moved to an out-of-home care facility.[139] According to Livingston, there are forty-four million people with dementia worldwide. This number is likely to double every twenty years. Those who care for such patients at home are seriously affected by this work, which is often performed out of love and is unpaid.[140]

Stress is a condition that everybody experiences and is as pervasive as the common cold. But different people respond differently to stress. One person's stressful situation can be a pleasurable experience for another person. The length and intensity of the stressor can impact individuals. In the case of those who care for patients with dementia, especially Alzheimer's, the impact can be exhausting and harmful.

Stress has been defined as a condition in which there is a discrepancy between the demands made upon a person and an individual's ability to respond to such a demand or pressure.[141] Caregivers can be in this kind of demanding situation for which they may have no easy way out, because in caring for loved ones, they often lack support. As the patient with Alzheimer's progressively becomes forgetful and unable to relate to others meaningfully, the challenge for the caregiver who should continue to give without any expectation becomes greater. Therefore, the presence, either in person or through other means of communication, of friends and relatives who support the caregiver becomes a vital necessity to prevent exhaustion and burnout.

Caregivers' stress may come from three sources: (1) from the fact that Alzheimer's is presently an incurable disease that is not possible to control and that has disabled someone who can't communicate properly; (2) from the repetitions and at times confusing behavior of the patient; and (3) from the inability of the caregivers to change the situation and have time to take care of themselves and meet their own personal needs due to of lack of support, human resources, financial means, and other difficulties. These can isolate the caregiver and cause discouragement and despair.

The above contributing factors generate a number of psychological reactions within the caregiver, such as anger directed toward the self and others, anxiety, depression, compassionate fatigue, exhaustion, and irritability. Moreover, social isolation, poor concentration, feelings of guilt, sleep problems, and stressful resentment may interfere with the daily tasks of caring. All of these underscore the need for support and counselling and for time off to relax, to restore energy and to reevaluate the situation in order to maintain good health and well-being.

In addition to psychological and emotional support, it has also been found helpful for caregivers to have a spiritual perspective in the process of treatment and caregiving. One benefit of prayer is that it enables one to realize that, after all, we are not masters of our destiny, nor are we in control of something that is uncontrollable. The sense of submission to the will of God Almighty who is the source of power and wisdom may bring comfort and solace to hearts and souls of those involved.

Having a spiritual perspective about life challenges and hardships can help to mitigate a sense of helplessness and despair. The following prayer used in AA group meetings is befitting: "God grant me serenity to accept the things I cannot change, courage to change the things I can, and wisdom to know the difference." Having faith and a broader perspective on life and a deeper understanding of its purpose and meaning may reduce the pain of a distressful situation. After all, the most helpless and vulnerable person in these circumstances is the patient, who did not ask to be sick with dementia.

When the body is exhausted, and the mind is unable to concentrate, it is time to ask for support and take a break. Meditation, exercise, being exposed to art and music, prayer, and a change of environment may help and make a difference. Sometimes reflecting on the relationship between the mind and the soul can give fresh inspiration. Happiness at the time of hardship is a gift: "Anybody can be happy in the state of comfort, ease, health, success, pleasure and joy; but if one will be happy and contented in the time of trouble, hardship and prevailing disease, it is the proof of nobility."[142]

Compassionate Fatigue and Caregivers

Compassionate fatigue is a condition that caregivers or family members of Alzheimer's patients may develop during the course of intensive and prolonged caring activities. Therefore, understanding the risk of compassionate fatigue among family members and professional caregivers of patients with Alzheimer's disease is important. According to Day and Anderson, there are many definitions of compassionate fatigue, but the most common one is this: "Compassionate fatigue is an adverse consequence of caring for individuals in need and the caregiver may experience the symptoms of anger, depression, and apathy.[143]

Family caregivers who look after relatives who are older adults with dementia on a full-time basis show symptoms of this condition of compassionate fatigue as well as anxiety, stress, feelings of resentment, hopelessness, and the fact that they have little free time for themselves. When these accumulate, they may lead to burnout and withdrawal from rendering service to these patients. Therefore, the family as a whole should be aware of the consequences of long-term caregiving and provide a well-planned working program for the caregivers to prevent compassionate fatigue and burnout by allowing sufficient time for caregivers to be free to attend to their own personal needs, rest, and, if needed, counseling.

There are many nursing homes for aged patients with Alzheimer's disease and other dementias, some operating as private and others as public facilities. Although in such places, efforts are made to make these patients feel comfortable, some families may feel reluctant to send their loved ones to such care centers, as they have the impression that they are abandoning the patient. However, there comes a time when an Alzheimer's patient requires day and night observation to ensure their well-being and security (e.g., patients may fall or injure themselves). Sadly, some of these nursing homes are short staffed and crowded, resulting in a decrease of compassionate care and a diminished positive attitude toward the patients. The following case reflects the challenge some individuals face in placing their parent in a nursing home.

My mother was diagnosed with Alzheimer's eight year ago. Five of the eight years she was able to live at home with my father and my sister. The past three years she has been in a nursing home…

We recently moved our mother to a different facility, one that offers an Alzheimer's unit with specialized care and a well-trained staff. Most nursing homes do not offer the proper kind of training for their staff to be able to deal effectively with an Alzheimer's patient. At the former health care facility she was in, their answer to everything was more medication, keep her doped up and she will be less trouble. They failed to realize that sleeping around the clock would cause her to become dehydrated, malnourished, as well as have urinary tract infections.

Moving our mother has been her salvation. The exclusiveness of the Alzheimer's unit has helped her to start having a better quality of life. Although the twinkle in her eye is fading, she still smiles and occasionally says a familiar name.[144] (Alzheimer's Association)

The above excerpt makes evident that with the rapid increase in the number of the Alzheimer's patients, there is a need for a system to insure that these vulnerable elderly patients receive proper care and are safe. This is an area of endeavor where governments, communities, and the medical establishment need to collaborate to significantly improve the situation. There is also a pressing need for proper care facilities for Alzheimer's patients as well as for trained staff and caregivers.

Spiritual Dimensions

As we age, we also think about our spirituality and having faith as a path to the future. But to some, the future is unknown and, therefore, there is nothing to look forward to after leaving this world. With this perspective, death and whatever lies beyond it is frightening. Physical and mental diseases such as dementia add to this fearsome view of the future. For some patients with Alzheimer's who don't believe in the spiritual aspects of life, the prospect of moving from the dark world of this disease to a dark world that is unknown and seemingly nonexistent can be terrifying.

Spirituality is a process, like a journey toward eternity, which is directed by a greater force, the divine reality. It is a journey toward God, during which we go through different stages, such as the stage of birth from the dark and confining world of the mother's womb. Then, after coming to this world of light and living in the matrix of the physical world, we then move to a new stage of evolution, and that is the spiritual world, where we will be free from the limitations of time and space and continue our journey in a new universe beyond our understanding in this world.

> Absolute repose does not exist in nature. All things either make progress or lose ground…"Progress" is the expression of spirit in the world of matter. The intelligence of man, his reasoning

powers, his knowledge, his scientific achievements, all these being manifestations of the spirit, partake of the inevitable law of spiritual progress and are, therefore, of necessity, immortal.[145]

Having such a vision stems from a belief in a creator. All religions have educated humankind that this world is a temporary one in which we develop our existential, mental, and spiritual capacities in order to be prepared for a new world beyond.

The human soul is part of our being what we are. It is not a material entity but rather is intangible. Therefore, it cannot be recognized in this material world. One may say it is like a vital force that acts through the instrumentation of the human brain to discover the mysteries of life and to bring about scientific, artistic, and creative development.

After the physical body, with all its organs (which serve as the instruments of the soul), comes to an end and dies, the soul takes its flight to the spiritual realm of the universe beyond. The soul or spirit does not die, as it is independent from the body and does not age as the body does. As mentioned earlier, its relationship with the body is like the relationship of the sun to a mirror. When the mirror breaks, the sun continues to exist. In other words, the evolution of the soul does not follow the development of the body, which is a biological organism that develops, ages, and then declines and finally dies and disintegrates. "Know thou that the soul of man is exalted above, and is independent of all infirmities of body or mind."[146]

What is the next world, and what are its characteristics? How does one prepare for it? 'Abdu'l-Bahá invites us to reflect on the following:

> That world beyond is a world of sanctity and radiance; therefore it is necessary that in this world he should acquire these divine attributes. In that world there is need of spirituality, faith, assurance, the knowledge and love of God. These he must attain

in this world so that after his ascension from the earthly to the heavenly Kingdom he shall find all that is needful in that life eternal ready for him...

...That divine world is manifestly a world of lights; therefore man has need of illumination here. That is a world of love; the love of God is essential. It is a world of perfections; virtues or perfections must be acquired. That world is vivified by the breaths of the Holy Spirit; in this world we must seek them. That is the Kingdom of life everlasting; it must be attained during this vanishing existence.[147]

To acquire spirituality, one must first possess faith, and to acquire faith, one needs to open one's heart to God and detach oneself from the vanities of this world and the defilement of earthly attachments. Spirituality is a phenomenon that has no boundaries. It seeks no status, no nationality, no linguistic barriers, and no gender differences. It discriminates against no race or color nor does it make a distinction between rich and poor. We don't need to have a university degree to qualify for spirituality. Sometimes wealth and even knowledge can become veils between individuals and their creator. This does not mean that knowledge is not needed; it is the cornerstone of civilization. But we also need faith.

The Aging Brain and the Human Soul

The brain is an instrument of the soul that develops its capacity but is also subject to the wear and tear of time and biological existence. It may eventually become degenerated and dysfunctional in extreme old age or as the result of disease. But the soul exists independently from this infirmity; it is eternal, as it is not a material entity and is thus free from the limitations of the material world and from disintegration and death.

> Know that the influence and perception of the human spirit is of two kinds; that is, the human spirit has two modes of operation and understanding. One mode is through the mediation of bodily instruments and organs. Thus it sees with the eye, hears with the ear, speaks with the tongue. These are actions of the spirit and operations of the human reality, but they occur through the mediation of bodily instruments…
>
> The other mode of the spirit's influence and action is without these bodily instruments and organs. For example, in the state of sleep, it sees without eyes, it hears without ears, it speaks without a tongue, it runs without feet—in brief, all these powers are exerted without the mediation of instruments and organs.[148]

In light of the above, it is quite possible that although patients with Alzheimer's disease lose their memory and intellectual faculties, they often maintain a sense of intuition and a mysterious spiritual awareness. This awareness, which they are unable to articulate, transcends the barrier of their illness.

In the Bahá'í writings, special emphasis has been put on the human spirit as a "divine trust." According to 'Abdu'l-Bahá, this divine trust "must traverse all conditions, for its passage and movement through the conditions of existence will be the means of its acquiring perfections."[149] Furthermore, He indicated that "The temple of man is like unto a mirror, his soul is as the sun, and his mental faculties even as the rays that emanate from that source of light. The ray may cease to fall upon the mirror, but it can in no wise be dissociated from the sun."[150] From this remark, we can discern that if mental faculties such as intelligence and memory (like the rays of the sun) become impaired, this by no means indicates that the soul has ceased to function; rather, it means that the instrument (the brain or mirror) is unable to reflect the power of those faculties. Likewise, if the computer breaks down, it is not an indication that the programmer has ceased to exist.

In the Bahá'í teachings, the relationship between mental illness and the human spirit is like the relationship between the cloud and the sun:

> Consider…the sun when it is completely hidden behind the clouds. Though the earth is still illumined with its light, yet the measure of light which it receiveth is considerably reduced. Not until the clouds have dispersed, can the sun shine again in the plenitude of its glory. Neither the presence of the cloud nor its absence can, in any way, affect the inherent splendor of the sun. The soul of man is the sun by which his body is illumined, and from which it draweth its sustenance, and should be so regarded.[151]

As the cloud prevents the sun from illuminating the earth, likewise mental illness prevents the soul from showing its power through the instrument of the body. The movement or the density of the clouds will have no effect on the natural quality of the sun, which is to shine. Likewise, the spirit is "changeless" and "indestructible."[152]

> Know thou that the soul of man is exalted above, and is independent of all infirmities of body or mind. That a sick person showeth signs of weakness is due to the hindrances that interpose themselves between his soul and his body, for the soul itself remaineth unaffected by any bodily ailments.[153]

Therefore, mental and physical illnesses have no bearing on the progress of the human spirit. The spirit will continue to advance, as progress is one of the essential qualities of the human spirit. Thus, it is conceivable that a person may suffer from mental or neurological illness and yet maintain his inherent spiritual capacity.

There are certain misunderstandings concerning the relationship between spirituality and human involvement in life crisis and environmental stress. One of these is the assumption that "being more spiritual" means having fewer problems to deal with or having no problems at all. But this is not the case. A person who conducts his or her life according to spiritual principles may have to face as many problems as anyone else. However, living one's life in such a way will enable one's capacity for tolerance and one's ability to accept stressful life events to grow along with a vision of life and its destiny.[154] Such a traveler on a long journey would realize that there might be unexpected surprises such as changes in climate, hazards of the road, unfriendly encounters, and new adaptations that have to be made to arrive at the destination. Crises would then be taken as new challenges for personal growth.

Some Suggestions on Caring

THE FOLLOWING ARE some additional thoughts and suggestions with respect to caring for patients with Alzheimer's disease:

- It will be important to reassess our attitude toward pain and suffering and to recognize the meaning of these difficulties in our personal growth and fulfillment. In a youth-worshipping and death-denying world, caring for old and aging people with or without dementia is a personal challenge that can give new meaning to our lives. It helps us grow and mature, and moves us away from our self-centeredness. To show love and care for someone who is helpless and impaired will help us develop the virtues of compassion and care that we need in our journey through this world. It will serve as an impetus for spiritual growth.
- It is necessary to accept patients as they are and not as they used to or ought to be. They cannot be changed by our wishes, but we can make life easier and safer for them. We must reflect and meditate on the nobility of the human soul in creation and respect this nobility under all conditions of the journey through this world. Illness is a condition that we do not choose; it comes to us as a part of life.
- Awareness that the elderly (especially patients with Alzheimer's disease) are frightened of rejection and of being abandoned

by their family members and friends is paramount. This view generates a great deal of anxiety and insecurity. Patients need to be reassured frequently that they will not be abandoned.

- Praying with the patient whenever possible is an activity that is positive both for the patient and the caregiver, if this is a practice they are comfortable with. The creative words of divine revelation are invested with a potency that can comfort the soul and alleviate pain and suffering, as they unfold the meaning and mystery of life before us. It is not always possible for a demented person to attend fully in reciting a prayer, but this does not mean that a person's soul is unaware of the prayerful moment spent with others.

- We may be able to discover certain clues that make contact with these patients more practical and possible. One seventy-eight-year-old patient was reported to show her delight only at the birthday of her grandchildren when she would spontaneously start singing "Happy Birthday." These precious moments were her only fleeting contact with the world of reality. After the birthday celebration, she would fade away and slip into her world of confusion.

- As long as possible, families should try to keep the patient at home in an accustomed environment in which he or she feels secure. The impersonal and sterile atmosphere of many professional institutions, in the absence of frequent family contact, can reinforce patients' belief that they are being abandoned. Care at home, however, is not always possible, as the advent of the terminal stage and the need for constant care, often for medical reasons, will make it necessary to give consideration to nursing homes or similar facilities. In some cultures, this separation can create a great deal of anguish and guilt in family members, while in other cultures such a decision is welcomed at a much earlier stage of the illness. It is a personal decision to be made at the family level, and it is never easy.

Conclusion

There is no doubt that memory and intellectual power are vital to our lives, and it is sad that a lifetime of knowledge and achievements should all fade away and disappear before our souls take flight to another world. How painful it is both for the person with Alzheimer's and their loved ones not to be able to say farewell to each other with clarity of mind prior to the death of such a patient.

The human mind is very complex, and the relationship between the intellect and the soul is far more mysterious and complicated than we can comprehend. Mental faculties have been described as property of the human soul.[155] Alzheimer's disease not only destroys brain cells, judgment, and memories, but it also seriously impairs marital or other close relationships.

If we dwell on the purely biological aspects of the degeneration of the brain that a person with Alzheimer's disease is suffering from, we may get frustrated at being unable to change the course of the illness, and our relationship with the patient may be affected in a negative way. On the other hand, if we fix our gaze beyond the neurological deterioration and focus on the spiritual being who is suffering from an illness that is outside of his or her understanding and control, we may be able to adopt a more positive and caring attitude.

Even if a treatment were to be discovered to delay the degeneration of brain cells, we would still need to maintain a caring attitude in providing comfort to these patients. Therefore, beyond all psychosocial and medical management efforts, we need to have faith and patience and honor the spiritual nature and nobility that makes up the essence of our humanness.

Caring and providing companionship for these helpless individuals is an invaluable service to this growing population. By spending time with such patients and alleviating their feelings of fear and estrangement, we, our families, and our children will learn new ways of relating to those who are progressively losing their intellectual faculties.

At the institutional level, governments, the medical system, the mental health establishment, and society at large need to develop a sustainable strategy to look after the aging population, including the increasing numbers of people suffering from Alzheimer's disease and other dementias. They will need to find creative ways to face this phenomenon and find a more humane approach while raising public awareness and understanding of this disease.

To those with grieving hearts who realize that their loved ones are progressively losing their memory through the ravages of Alzheimer's disease, the following words of 'Abdu'l-Bahá to Professor Auguste Forel, a renowned scientific figure, may bring some comfort: "Consider how the human intellect develops and weakens, and may at times come to naught, whereas the soul changeth not."[156]

In conclusion, while we are still on our journey in this world, we should prepare ourselves by acquiring divine virtues, among which are love of humanity, kindness and compassion, spirituality, faith, assurance, and the knowledge and love of our creator. These are essential for the progress of our souls.

When our thoughts are filled with the bitterness of this world,
let us turn our eyes to the sweetness of God's compassion and

He will send us heavenly calm! If we are imprisoned in the material world, our spirit can soar into the Heavens and we shall be free indeed!

When our days are drawing to a close let us think of the eternal worlds, and we shall be full of joy![157]

REFERENCES

1. B. D. McPherson. *Ageing as a Social Process* (Toronto: Harcourt Canada, 1998), 10–12.
2. Ibid., 10–12.
3. Ibid., 38.
4. Ibid., 38.
5. Ibid., 40.
6. Ibid., 33.
7. UNDESA, World Population Ageing 2011, World Population Prospects, 2010 Revision.
8. A-M. Ghadirian, *Ageing: Challenges and Opportunities* (Oxford: George Ronald, 1991), 112.
9. R. Suzman and J. Beard, *Global Health and Aging—WHO National Institute on Aging, Overview*, March 9, 2012, 2, http://who.int/ageing/publications/global_health.pdf?ua=1
10. "World Population Prospects: The 2010 Revision," United Nations, http://esa.un.org/unpd/wpp
11. Suzman, op. cit., 2.
12. Ibid.
13. G. Small, "Alzheimer's disease and other dementing disorders," in *Comprehensive Textbook of Psychiatry*, 6th ed. (Baltimore: Williams and Wilkins, 1995), 2. 2562.

14 W. Xu, C. Ferrari and H-W. Wang, "Epidemiology of Alzheimer's Disease", in *Understanding Alzheimer's Disease*, ed. Inga Zerr, February 27, 2013, http:/www.intechopen.com./books/understanding-alzheimer-s-disease/epidemiology-of-alzheimer-s-disease, 330.

15 Leon J. Thal, "Dementia Update: Diagnosis and Neuropsychiatric Aspects," *Journal of Clinical Psychiatry* (supplement) 49:5 (May 1988).

16 R. W. Banchard and M. N. Rossor, "Typical clinical features (dementia)," in *Clinical Diagnosis and Management of Alzheimer's Disease* (Martin Dunitz Ltd., 1996), 35–48.

17 American Psychiatric Association, *Diagnostic and Statistical Manual of Mental Disorders*, 3rd ed. (Washington, DC: American Psychiatric Press Inc., 1987), 107.

18 R. Preidt, "Alzheimer's cases expected to double by 2050, researchers say," Medline Plus, November 14, 2014, http://www.nlm.nih.gov/medlineplus/news/fullstory_149464.html Health Day 2014 http://www.healthday.com.

19 D. E. Barnes and K. Yaffe, "The projected effect of risk factor reduction on Alzheimer's disease prevalence," *The Lancet Neurology*, 10, no. 9, September 2011, 819–828.

20 F. Massoud and G. C. Leger, "Pharmacological Treatment of Alzheimer Disease," *The Canadian Journal of Psychiatry* 56, no. 10 (October 2011): 579–588.

21 C. P. Ferri et al. "Global prevalence of dementia: a Delphi consensus study," *Lancet* (2005);366(9503): 2112–2117.

22 C. Qiu, M. Kivipelto, and E. Strauss, "Epidemiology of Alzheimer's disease: occurrence, determinants, and strategies toward intervention," *Dialogues Clin Neurosci* (2009);11:111–128.

23 A. Levin, "Kandel details brain's role in growth and loss of memory," *American Psychiatric News* (July 18, 2014): 26.

24 "Alzheimer's Disease Fact Sheet, National Institute of Aging (NIH-US)," December 12, 2014, http://www.nia.nih.gov/alzheimers/publication/alzheimers-disease-fact-sheet.

25 Xu et al., op.cit., 334.

26 J. Blass and J. Poirier, "Pathophysiology of the Alzheimer syndrome" in *Clinical Diagnosis and Management of Alzheimer's Disease.* (London: Martin Duritz Ltd., 1996), 17–20.

27 D. Kwon, "Evidence for person-to-person transmission of Alzheimer's pathology," *Scientific American, Health*, September 9, 2015, http://www.scientificamerican.com/article/evidence-for-person-to-person-transmission-of-alzheimer-s-pathology.

28 J. Hoffman, S. Froemke, and S. K. Golant, *The Alzheimer's Project—Momentum in Science. Based on the HBO Documentary Book* (New York: Tree Public Affairs, 2009), 136.

29 Ibid., 133–135.

30 Ibid., 133–135.

31 Ibid., 134–135.

32 Ibid., 135.

33 J. Ingram, *The End of Memory* (Toronto: Harper Collins Publishers Ltd., 2014), 95.

34 N. Doidge, *The Brain that Changes Itself* (New York: Penguin Books, 2007), 253–257.

35 Alzheimer Society of Canada, "Changes in the brain," January 20, 2014, http://www.alzheimer.ca/en/About-dementia/Alzheimer-s-disease/What-is-Alzheimer-s-disease/Changes-in-the-brain.

36 M. S. Wolfe, "Shutting Down Alzheimer's," *Scientific American* (May 2006), 73.

37 Ibid.

38 A. M. Ghadirian, *Creative Dimensions of Suffering* (Wilmette, IL: Bahá'í Publishing, 2009), 85–100.

39. B. Brownstein, "Julianne Moore Triumphs," *Montreal Gazette*, January 23, 2015.
40. J. M. Nash, "The new science of Alzheimer's," *Time*, July 17, 2000, 33.
41. N. L. Mace and P. V. Rabins, *The 36-Hour Day* (Baltimore: The John Hopkins University Press, 1981), 119.
42. Ibid., 120.
43. Hoffman et al., op. cit., 58–59.
44. G. He et al. "Gamma-secretase activating protein is a therapeutic target for Alzheimer's disease," *Nature* 467 (September 2, 2010), 95–98, http://www.nature.com/nature/journal/v467/n7311/full/nature09325.html
45. S. Karceski "Preventing Alzheimer disease with exercise?" *Neurology.* (April 24, 2012);78(17):e110-2, http://www.neurology.org/content/78/17/e110.full.pdf.
46. Hoffman et al., op. cit., 54.
47. Ibid., 58–59.
48. K. M. Robinson, "5 myths about Alzheimer's Disease," WebMD LLC, January 23, 2015, http://www.webmd.com/alzheimers/features/5-alzheimers-disease-myths.
49. Ibid.
50. "Alzheimer's myths," Alzheimer's Association, October 24, 2015, http:/www.alz.org/alzheimers_disease_myths_about_alzheimers.asp.
51. Ibid.
52. "Warning Signs," Alzheimer Society of Canada http://www.alzheimer.ca/en/About-dementia/Alzheimer-s-disease/Warning-signs-and-symptoms/10-warning-signs.
53. Xu et al., op. cit., 335.
54. Blass and Poirier, "Pathophysiology of the Alzheimer syndrome," op. cit., 20.

55. D. E. Barnes and K. Yaffe, "The projected effect of risk factor reduction on Alzheimer's disease prevalence," op. cit., 819–828.
56. Xu et al., op. cit., 337.
57. V. Watts, "Cognitive decline may begin as early as young adulthood," *Psychiatric News* 28 (February 6, 2015).
58. Xu et al., op. cit., 337.
59. Ibid., 338.
60. M. Olfson, M. King, and M. Schoenbaum, "Benzodiazepine use in the United States," *JAMA Psychiatry* (December 17, 2014), archpsycjamanetwork.com/article.aspx?articleid=2019955.
61. "Despite Risks, Benzodiazepine Use Highest in Older People," DocGuide.com, December 17, 2014, http://www.docguide.com/despite-risks-benzodiazepine-use-highest-older-people?tsid=5.
62. Ibid.
63. S. Billoti de Gage et al., " Benzodiazepine use and risk of Alzheimer's disease: case-control study," *British Medical Journal* 349 (September 9, 2014), 349: 5205, http://www.bmj.com/content/349/bmj.g5205.
64. "Despite Risks, Benzodiazepine Use Highest in Older People," op. cit., December 17, 2014.
65. B. Mander, "Alzheimer's-linked brain proteins tied to poor sleep in study," US National Library of Medicine, June 1, 2015, http://www.nlm.nih.gov/medlineplus/news/fullstory_152838.html.
66. "Sleep Disturbance Linked to Amyloid in Brain Area Affected by Alzheimer's Disease," Doctor's Guide, December 9, 2014, http://www.docguide.org/news/content.nsf/news/18FFA68331BDC61485257DA900719E8F.
67. Ibid.
68. Xu et al., op. cit., 339.
69. Ibid., 338.

70 S. Rovio et al. "Leisure-time physical activity at midlife and the risk of dementia and Alzheimer's disease." *Lancet Neurol* 4 no. 11 (2005):705–711.
71 Hoffman et al., op. cit., 150.
72 M. Dezell and C. Hill, *The Everything Health Guide to Alzheimer's Disease* (Avon, MA: Adams Media, 2009).
73 "Healthy diet may help shield the aging brain," US National Library of Medicine, MedlinePlus, July 23, 2015, http://www.nlm.nih.gov/medlineplus/news/fullstory_153742.html.
74 Ibid., 152.
75 Ibid.
76 M. C. Morris et al. "Dietary fats and the risk of incident Alzheimer disease." *Arch Neurol* 60, no. 2 (2003):194–200.
77 C. De Jage, "Omega 3 levels affect whether B vitamins can slow cognitive decline," *DG News*, January 19, 2016, http://dgnews.docguide.com/omega-3-levels-affect-whether-b-vitamins-can-slow-cognitive-decline.
78 Hoffman et al., op. cit., 152–153.
79 B. Vellas et al, "Long-term use of standardised ginkgo biloba extract for the prevention of Alzheimer's disease (GuidAge): a randomised placebo-controlled trial." *Lancet Neurology*, September 6, 2012, http://www.ncbi.nlm.nih.gov/pubmed/22959217.
80 M. H. Eskelinen and M. Kivipleto, "Caffeine as a protective factor in dementia and Alzheimer's disease," *J. Alzheimer's disease* (2010); 20 Suppl. 1:S167–74. doi: 10.3233/JAD-2010–1404.
81 Doidge, op. cit., 253–257.
82 Ibid., 254.
83 Ibid., 255.
84 "Exercise may buffer symptoms of early Alzheimer's," US National Library of Medicine, MedlinePlus: July 23, 2015, http://www.nlm.nih.gov/medlineplus/news/fullstory_153739.html.

85 Ibid.
86 Levin, op. cit. 26.
87 Ibid.
88 Qiu et al., op. cit., 111–128.
89 J. Arehart-Treichel, "Several factors may counter prediction of Alzheimer's crisis," *American Psychiatric News*, April 18, 2008, 25.
90 Ibid., 25.
91 Hoffman et al., op. cit. 138–139.
92 Xu et al., op. cit., 340.
93 Hoffman et al., op. cit., 138.
94 J. Arehart-Treichel, "Cognitive impairment affects 1 in 5 elderly Americans," *American Psychiatric News* 25, April 18, 2008.
95 T. Haelle, "Many U.S. households include someone with failing memory," *HealthDay News*, March 5, 2015, http://consumer.healthday.com/cognitive-health-information-26/alzheimer-s-news-20/many-u-s-households-include-someone-with-failing-memory-697144.html.
96 N. D. Anderson, K. J. Murphy, and A. K. Troyer, *Living with Mild Cognitive Impairment* (Toronto: Oxford University Press, 2012), 30–31.
97 Ibid., 31.
98 Ibid., 4.
99 American Psychiatric Association, *Alzheimer's Disease. Let's Talk about Mental Illness* (Washington, DC: American Psychiatric Press Inc., 1992).
100 Anderson et al., op. cit.p. 7.
101 Ibid., 26.
102 Ibid., 27.
103 S. J. Crutch, R. Isaacs, and M. N. Rossor, "Some workmen can blame their tools: artistic change in an individual with Alzheimer's disease," *The Lancet* 357 (June 30, 2001): 2129–2133.

104 Ibid.
105 B. L. Miller, cited by S. Jeffrey, "How some declining dementia patients gain creative abilities," *The Medical Post*, Canadian edition (September 14, 1998): 46.
106 B. L. Miller et al., "Enhanced artistic activity with temporal lobe degeneration," *Lancet* 348 (1996): 1744–55.
107 S. M. Koger, K. Chapin, and M. Brotons, "Is music therapy an effective intervention for dementia? A meta-analytic review of literature," (Abstract) *Journal of Music Therapy*, American Music Therapy Association (1998).
108 Miller, cited by Jeffrey, "How some declining dementia patients gain creative abilities," op., cit., 46.
109 B. L. Miller et al., "Functional correlates of musical and visual ability in frontotemporal dementia," *British Journal of Psychiatry* 176 (2000): 459.
110 R. Preidt: "Singing hits a high note for folks with early dementia," *Health Day, Medline Plus*, December 17, 2015, https://www.nlm.nih.gov/medlineplus/news/fullstory_156287.html.
111 A-M. Ghadirian, *Creative Dimensions of Suffering*, op. cit., 83–100.
112 C. H. Espinel, "Memory and the Creation of Art: The Syndrome, as in de Kooning, of 'Creating in the Midst of Dementia,'" in "Neurological Disorders in Famous Artists—Part 2," *Front Neurol Neurosci*. 22 (Basel: Karger, 2007): 150–168.
113 S. Gauthier, *Clinical Diagnosis and Management of Alzheimer's Disease*, (London: Martin Duritz Ltd., 1996), 205–267.
114 A. F. Schatzberg and C. De Battista, *Manual of Clinical Psychopharmacology*, 8th edition (Washington, DC: American Psychiatric Publishing, 2015), 665–669.
115 Ibid.
116 Ibid.
117 Gauthier, op cit., 205–267.

118 Koger and M. Brotons: "Is Music Therapy an Effective Intervention for Dementia?" op. cit.
119 "News & Notes: Families Provide Bulk of Care to Persons with Alzheimer's Disease and Other Dementias." *Hospital and Community Psychiatry* 35, no. 9, September 1987.
120 'Abdu'l-Bahá, *Tablet to Auguste Forel, The Bahá'í World*, Vol. XV, Bahá'í World Centre, Haifa, 1976, 8–9.
121 Alzheimer's Association, July 4, 2015, http://www.alz.org/living_with_alzheimers_8711.asp.
122 Alzheimer's Caregiving Tips: Changes in Intimacy and Sexuality, July 2012, www.nia.nih.gov/alzheimers /topics/caregiving.
123 *Lights of Guidance: A Bahá'í Reference File*, 6th ed. (New Delhi: Bahá'í Publishing Trust, 1999), #768, 231.
124 B. D. McPherson, op. cit., 33–34.
125 Ibid., 209–210.
126 Ibid., 38.
127 S. Mahieu and C. A. Cohen, *Support of families. In Clinical Diagnosis and Management of Alzheimer's Disease*, S. Gauthier (ed) (London: Martin Dunitz Ltd., 1996), 294.
128 Alzheimer's Association, http://www.alz.org/living_with_alzheimers_10594.asp.
129 Hong Li et al., "Caring burden and associated factors of care providers for senile dementia patients in an urban-rural fringe of Fuzhou City, China," *Aging Clin Exp Res* 24, no. 6 (2012): 712.
130 Ibid., 710.
131 Ibid., 707–713.
132 Alzheimer's Association, July 4, 2015, http://www.alz.org/living_with_alzheimers_10300.asp.
133 Psychosocial intervention for adult-child caregivers of parents with Alzheimer's disease, National Institute on Aging, July 31, 2015, https://www.nia.nih.gov/alzheimers/clinical-trials/

psychosocial-intervention-adult-child-caregivers-parents-alzheimers.
134 'Abdu'l-Bahá, *Some Answered Questions*. Collected and translated from the Persian by Laura Clifford Barney. Revised. (Haifa: Bahá'í World Centre, 2014), 267.
135 Shoghi Effendi, cited in Lights of Guidance, 231, 6th edition, 1999.
136 Universal House of Justice, letter of December 18, 2014.
137 *World Alzheimer Report 2013*, London, UK, Alzheimer's Disease International, 2013, chapter 6, 26.
138 S. H. Zarit, N. K. Orr, and J. M. Zarit, *The Hidden Victims of Alzheimer's Disease* (New York: New York Press, 1985).
139 G. Livingston et al., "Long-term clinical and cost-effectiveness of psychological intervention for family carers of people with dementia: a single-blind, randomized controlled trial," *The Lancet Psychiatry* 1, no. 7 (November 2014): 539–548.
140 Ibid.
141 G. Caplan, "Mastery of stress: Psychosocial aspects," *American Journal of Psychiatry* 138, no. 4 (April 1981): 414.
142 'Abdu'l-Bahá, *Baha'i World Faith* (Wilmette, IL: Bahá'í Publishing Trust, 1976), 363.
143 J. R. Day and R. A. Anderson, "Compassionate fatigue: An application of the concept of informal caregivers of family members with dementia." *Nursing Research and Practice* (September 8, 2011). Online article on website: http://www.ncbi.nlm.nih.gov/pmc/articles/PMC3170786/
144 www.alz.org/living_with_alzheimers_10236.asp, July 4, 2015.
145 'Abdu'l-Bahá, *Paris Talks*, 88.
146 Bahá'u'lláh, *Gleanings from the Writings of Bahá'u'lláh*, trans. Shoghi Effendi (Wilmette, IL.: Bahá'í Publishing Trust, 1983), 153–54.

[147] 'Abdu'l-Bahá, *Foundations of World Unity* (Wilmette, IL: Bahá'í Publishing Trust, 1945), 63–64.
[148] 'Abdu'l-Bahá, *Some Answered Questions*, op. cit., 2014 edition, 261.
[149] Ibid., 200.
[150] 'Abdu'l-Bahá, *Tablet to Auguste Forel*, op. cit., *Bahá'í World XV*, 43.
[151] Bahá'u'lláh, *Gleanings from the Writings of Bahá'u'lláh*, op. cit. p.155.
[152] 'Abdu'l-Bahá, *Paris Talks*. London: Bahá'í Publishing Trust, 1995, p.65.
[153] Bahá'u'lláh, *Gleanings*, op. cit. pp.153–54.
[154] Ghadirian, A-M. *Ageing: Challenges and Opportunities*. Oxford, George Ronald, 1991. 110–118.
[155] 'Abdu'l-Bahá, *Tablet to August Forel*, op. cit., 38.
[156] Ibid.
[157] 'Abdu'l-Bahá, *Paris Talks*, op. cit., 111.

Author Biography

Dr. A-M. Ghadirian is a physician and professor emeritus on the faculty of medicine at McGill University in Montreal, Canada. For twenty-four years, he served as director of the Royal Victoria Hospital's mood disorders clinic, where he researched the psychological and biological aspects of psychiatric disorders.

He has over 140 publications, including scientific articles in peer-reviewed journals, chapters in books, and research works on aging, memory dysfunction, and Alzheimer's disease. A few of his most recent works include *Creative Dimensions of Suffering*, *Materialism: Moral and Social Consequences*, and *Steadfastness in the Covenant*.

Dr. Ghadirian is a Distinguished Life Fellow of the American Psychiatric Association and recipient of the Association of Universities and Colleges of Canada's Senior Scholar Award and the Association of Baha'i Studies's Distinguished Scholarship Award, among others.

He earned his MSc degree in psychiatry in the United States and received advanced training at McGill University.

His website address is: www.medicineandspirituality.com